The
Crohn's Disease
and
Ulcerative Colitis
Fact Book

The
Crohn's Disease
and
Ulcerative Colitis
Fact Book

National Foundation for Ileitis & Colitis

edited by

Peter A. Banks, M.D.; Daniel H. Present, M.D.;
and Penny Steiner, M.P.H.

CHARLES SCRIBNER'S SONS
NEW YORK

Copyright © 1983 National Foundation for Ileitis & Colitis, Inc.

Library of Congress Cataloging in Publication Data

Main entry title:

The Crohn's disease and ulcerative colitis fact book.

Includes bibliographical references and index.
1. Enteritis, Regional. 2. Ulcerative colitis.
I. Banks, Peter A. II. Present, Daniel H. III. Steiner, Penny. IV. National Foundation for Ileitis & Colitis (U.S.) [DNLM: 1. Crohn's disease. 2. Colitis, Ulcerative. WI 522 C9412
RC862.E52C77   1983   616.3'44   83-11602
ISBN 0-684-17967-9

1 3 5 7 9 11 13 15 17 19 F/C 20 18 16 14 12 10 8 6 4 2

Printed in the United States of America.

CONTRIBUTING
AUTHORS

Arthur H. Aufses, Jr., M.D.
Mount Sinai Medical Center
New York, New York

Benjamin M. Banks, M.D.
Beth Israel Hospital
Boston, Massachusetts

Naomi Banks, M.B.A.
Boston, Massachusetts

Peter A. Banks, M.D.
St. Elizabeth's Hospital
Beth Israel Hospital
Boston, Massachusetts

Leslie H. Bernstein, M.D.
Montefiore Medical Center
Bronx, New York

Lawrence J. Brandt, M.D.
Montefiore Medical Center
Bronx, New York

Leonard Katz, M.D.
State University of New York
(Buffalo)
School of Medicine
Buffalo, New York

Barbara S. Kirschner, M.D.
University of Chicago Hos-
pitals and Clinics
Chicago, Illinois

Burton I. Korelitz, M.D.
Lenox Hill Hospital
New York, New York

J. Thomas LaMont, M.D.
Boston University Medical
Center
Boston, Massachusetts

Albert I. Mendeloff, M.D.
Sinai Hospital of Baltimore
Baltimore, Maryland

v

CONTRIBUTING AUTHORS

Stanley Meltzer, Esq.
New York, New York

Michael L. Miller, C.L.U.
New York, New York

Daniel H. Present, M.D.
Mount Sinai Medical Center
New York, New York

Jane W. Present, M.A.
Trustee, NFIC
New York, New York

James M. Rabb, M.D.
Beth Israel Hospital
St. Elizabeth's Hospital
Boston, Massachusetts

George B. Rankin, M.D.
Cleveland Clinic Foundation
Cleveland, Ohio

Arvey I. Rogers, M.D.
Veterans Administration
  Medical Center
Miami, Florida

Suzanne Rosenthal
Executive Vice-President, NFIC
New York, New York

David B. Sachar, M.D.
Mount Sinai Medical Center
New York, New York

Jay B. Shumaker, M.D.
Tufts University Medical School
Boston, Massachusetts

Milton Singer, M.D.
St. Barnabas Medical Center
Livingston, New Jersey

Penny Steiner, M.P.H.
Education & Publications
  Director, NFIC
New York, New York

Walter R. Thayer, M.D.
Rhode Island Hospital
Providence, Rhode Island

Jerome Waye, M.D.
Mount Sinai Medical Center
New York, New York

Maurice J. Zimmerman, M.D.
Mount Sinai Medical Center
New York, New York

CONTENTS

Foreword   *ix*

Preface   *xi*

Part I. *The Nature of the Diseases*

1. Definitions   *1*
2. Who Gets Crohn's Disease and Ulcerative Colitis?   *12*
3. What Causes Crohn's Disease and Ulcerative Colitis?   *19*
4. Diagnosing Crohn's Disease and Ulcerative Colitis   *28*
5. Systemic Manifestations   *44*

Part II. *Treating the Diseases*

6. Medications and Their Side Effects   *55*

7. Nutritional Complications of Crohn's Disease
   and Ulcerative Colitis   71
8. The Role of Surgery   82
9. The Threat of Cancer   97

Part III. *Living with the Diseases*

10. Crohn's Disease and Ulcerative Colitis in
    Children   109
11. Pregnancy   120
12. Crohn's Disease and Ulcerative Colitis in
    Older People   125
13. The Role of the Emotions   131
14. Coping with Hospitalization   137
15. Obtaining Life Insurance and Medical
    Insurance   145
16. What to Do if You Become Disabled   152

Appendix: NFIC Directory of Chapters   159
Notes   163
Glossary   171
Index   185

FOREWORD

The National Foundation for Ileitis & Colitis has long recognized the need for a complete reference book for patients with Crohn's disease and ulcerative colitis. Patients who understand the natural course and best management of their disease are less frustrated by its complications and better able to tolerate the effects of illness and treatments. Informed patients also raise the consciousness of the medical community, enabling their doctors to learn more about the best possible treatments for them.

The authors and editors faced many challenges in the preparation of this book, most of them the result of our ignorance of the cause of Crohn's disease and ulcerative colitis. [As long as the cause remains unknown,] specific treatment must await this further knowledge. Current "facts" consist of creative research, clinical experience, and hard-won, extensive observation. Today, in 1983, the number of observers has increased and the experience has multiplied accordingly. The National Foundation for Ileitis & Colitis, with its vigorous program of research, has made most of this possible.

With increasing experience comes a diversity in approach to the diseases. Special effort has been made by the editors to balance these differences in approach, so that the reader is presented with the most accurate appraisal of what we now know about Crohn's disease and ulcerative colitis.

I congratulate the authors and editors and convey to them the deep appreciation of NFIC's National Scientific Advisory Committee for this publication which patients and their physicians have so long awaited.

Burton I. Korelitz, M.D.
Chairman, National Scientific Advisory Committee
National Foundation for Ileitis & Colitis

PREFACE

Crohn's disease and ulcerative colitis are not easy diseases to deal with. They're not easy for the physician to diagnose and treat, and they're certainly not easy for people who must cope with their symptoms every day. When the National Foundation for Ileitis & Colitis (NFIC) was founded in 1967 as a partnership of physicians and patients, one of its paramount goals was to dispel the appalling ignorance surrounding this pair of little-known, little-talked-about digestive diseases. Today, despite NFIC's energetic efforts to educate and inform the public, there are still physicians who know little about the diseases, and patients who remain ignorant and afraid because no one has told them what to expect. This is the reason for this book.

The editors wish to thank the many physicians and laypersons associated with the foundation who have contributed the chapters in this book, and the NFIC staff members who helped in preparing the manuscript. Each one has brought special knowledge and dedication to the task. Because of their efforts, we have been able to assemble the most up-to-date information about Crohn's disease and ulcerative colitis, which we hope has been expressed in a readable, understandable fashion. This is no small accomplishment with diseases and symptoms that are unfashionable and frustratingly difficult to treat.

For those individuals and families who must live with these illnesses from day to day, we hope that this book will become a trusted companion, a resource that will clear away the mysteries and make living with Crohn's disease and ulcerative colitis a little easier.

Peter A. Banks, M.D.
Daniel H. Present, M.D.
Penny Steiner, M.P.H.

PART I

The Nature of the Diseases

1

DEFINITIONS

What are Crohn's disease and ulcerative colitis? A great deal of confusion surrounds the many medical terms used to describe these illnesses. Some of these words have changed over the years as knowledge about the disease has increased and old terms have been replaced by new ones. The following definitions should help clear away some of the confusion and acquaint you with the latest terminology.

ulcerative colitis — Inflammation and ulceration of the inner lining of the large intestine (colon) and rectum (Figure 1). When this inflammation is confined to the rectum alone it is called ulcerative proctitis. Ulcerative colitis is *not* the same as spastic colitis, which is an incorrect term used to describe irritable bowel syndrome. Ulcerative colitis is a serious disease; irritable bowel syndrome is not.
Crohn's disease — an inflammatory disease that attacks the lower (distal) small intestine (ileitis), the colon (Crohn's disease of the colon, Crohn's colitis, granulomatous colitis), or

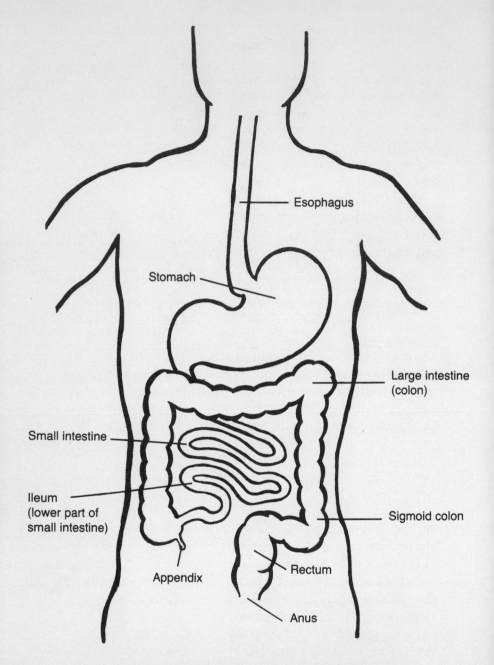

Esophagus

Stomach

Large intestine
(colon)

Small intestine

Ileum
(lower part of
small intestine)

Sigmoid colon

Appendix

Rectum

Anus

Figure 1. Diagram of the stomach and intestines.

both small intestine and colon (ileocolitis). In the early years following its discovery, Crohn's disease was called *regional ileitis* or *regional enteritis,* since physicians observed that the inflammation was patchy and skipped over areas of healthy bowel. Today, the term *Crohn's disease* (named for its co-discoverer, Burrill B. Crohn, M.D.) has replaced the use of these older terms.

Both Crohn's disease and ulcerative colitis may cause diarrhea, abdominal pain, rectal bleeding, and fever. Decreased appetite and weight loss are common. The diseases may begin slowly or develop quite suddenly, and can produce a range of symptoms that affect the whole body. The diseases are chronic, and as yet their cause—and therefore their cure—are unknown. Some people have mild symptoms while others have severe and disabling ones. Medications currently available decrease inflammation and control symptoms but do not provide a cure. Because the symptoms and complications of Crohn's disease and ulcerative colitis are so similar, the two diseases are grouped together under the name inflammatory bowel disease (IBD). The abbreviation IBD will be used throughout this book to refer conveniently to both diseases.

RULING OUT OTHER PROBLEMS

Before a diagnosis of IBD can be made, it is necessary for the physician to rule out the presence of other serious and not-so-serious bowel disorders with similar symptoms. First, there are a variety of infections caused by specific organisms that produce symptoms mimicking Crohn's disease or ulcerative colitis. These include infections caused by two intestinal parasites: *E. histolytica,* which causes amebic dysentery of the colon (amebiasis), and *Giardia lamblia,* which causes a chronic diarrheal disorder of the upper small intestine (giardiasis). Another group of disorders is caused by bacteria of the shigella, salmonella, yersinia, and campylobacter families. Shigella causes inflammation of the colon, which closely resembles ulcerative colitis; the other three bacteria may cause inflammation of either the lower ileum or the colon which looks very much like Crohn's disease. These infectious agents can be identified by appropriate examinations of the stool and in the case of giardiasis, by collecting fluid samples from the upper small intestine.

Second, we now know that a variety of antibiotics may suppress the growth of normal bacteria in the colon and permit the overgrowth of a species of bacteria in the clostridium family. These organisms produce a toxin that may cause severe diarrhea and at times severe colitis. This antibiotic-associated colitis may closely resemble ulcerative colitis. Fortunately, there is a specific examination of the stool which can reliably identify the presence of this toxin within forty-eight hours. Fortunately also, there are several antibiotics that can be used to eradicate the clostridia responsible for this illness and thereby cure the inflammation.

In addition, there are several "functional" disorders of the bowel that cause symptoms very much like those of IBD. These disorders are currently given the name irritable bowel syndrome (IBS), but have also been called (incorrectly) spastic colitis, mucous colitis, and "nervous stomach." Unlike Crohn's disease and ulcerative colitis, these disorders do not cause inflammation of the bowel wall. The colon is normal to microscopic examination and infectious agents have not been identified in this disorder. Barium enema and upper gastrointestinal (GI) X rays do not show significant abnormalities. Researchers feel that IBS may be caused by abnormalities in bowel motility (called peristalsis) ranging from very inactive to overactive. Diarrhea and constipation may occur in the same patient at different times. While the basic cause of IBS has not been found, there is frequently a correlation with life stresses or with poor adaptation to these stresses. Recent studies have also shown sensitivity to certain foods. The important points to emphasize are that irritable bowel syndrome is different from inflammatory bowel disease, does not cause any inflammatory process in the body, and does not develop into IBD.

ULCERATIVE COLITIS

Ulcerative colitis is an inflammatory disease of the colon and rectum. When the disease process is limited to the rectum, it is called ulcerative proctitis. If it involves only the rectum and sigmoid colon, it is termed *ulcerative proctosigmoiditis*. These are less serious forms of ulcerative colitis. In addition to the rectum and sigmoid colon, ulcerative colitis may involve a larger portion of colon or even the entire colon. Two points should be emphasized here. In ulcerative colitis, the rectum is almost always inflamed at the onset of illness. This often helps in distinguishing the disease from Crohn's disease of the colon, in which the rectum is frequently normal and a portion of the colon above the rectum may be inflamed. The second point is that the disease is continous and not patchy in the area involved. For example, if the disease involves the rectum, sigmoid colon, and transverse colon, these areas are uniformly involved without intervening normal areas.

The first sign of ulcerative colitis or proctitis is usually the passage of stools which are softer and looser than normal. Blood is usually mixed with the stool. Some patients may feel the urgent need to defecate (tenesmus) which is localized in the rectum and is occasionally severe enough to result in accidental soiling. This is caused by rectal inflammation and may be relieved temporarily by the passage of a small amount of liquid stool mixed with blood and secretions. Unfortunately, within a few minutes or a few hours, the extreme urgency to move the bowels returns. This need for frequent evacuation may also occur at night and may interfere with sleep. In addition to tenesmus, it is common to feel cramping abdominal pain caused by inflammation in other parts of the colon. This pain is often relieved by moving the bowels.

The diagnosis of ulcerative colitis is usually made on the basis of clinical findings combined with two tests: sigmoidoscopy and barium enema X ray. These will be discussed in Chapter 4.

The course of chronic ulcerative colitis is variable. In many cases, symptoms are not very severe, there are no systemic manifestations (such as joint pains, or skin and eye inflammations), and the patient does not lose weight or have difficulty other than the frequent passage of stool mixed with blood. This is most common when the involvement is limited to the rectum and sigmoid colon. Despite what may look like excessive bleeding, persons with this localized form of the disease rarely become anemic. An important point to make is that when the inflammation is limited initially to the rectum, only rarely does it spread at a later time to involve other portions of the colon. When the involvement does spread to other portions of the colon or when most of the colon is involved from the start, symptoms tend to be more severe and include weakness, anemia caused by rectal bleeding, crampy abdominal pain, fever, and weight loss. Nevertheless, ulcerative colitis is a disease characterized by remissions as well as by exacerbations. Remissions are periods in which the disease is quiescent and the patient experiences few or no symptoms. Exacerbations mean symptomatic flare-ups or increased inflammation. During remissions, ulcerations heal, and the lining of the colon may return to normal or near normal as demonstrated by sigmoidoscopy, barium enema, colonoscopy, and even biopsies of the colon.

A remission may be either spontaneous or induced by medication. (Chapter 6 describes the medications currently used to treat IBD.) Even when a remission lasts for a long time and the colon appears to return completely to normal, physicians do not call this a cure, since the disease may flare up at any time. Many patients are treated successfully with medications during each exacerbation and are not overly handicapped by their ulcerative colitis. However, the small percentage of patients whose symptoms are very severe or relentless, or cases where there is a strong suspicion of cancer of the colon may require complete surgical removal of the colon and rectum (proctocolectomy). At the present time, this is the only known cure for ulcerative colitis.

ULCERATIVE PROCTITIS

Ulcerative proctitis is a mild form of ulcerative colitis confined to the rectum and characterized by intermittent bleeding in the stool. The bowel pattern is often normal, but occasional diarrhea or constipation is not unusual. Discharge of mucus may accompany bleeding. Tenesmus caused by inflammation in the rectum may also be troublesome. Generalized symptoms, such as fever, weight loss, and weakness, are rare.

Fortunately, this form of colitis seldom extends to involve a larger portion of the colon. A striking feature of ulcerative proctitis is the clear separation of the abnormal portion from the normal bowel above it. When the physician examines the rectum and lower colon using the sigmoidoscope, the inflammation will usually be found to extend 10 centimeters or so into the rectum. Above that, the colon looks completely normal, and biopsies and X-ray examinations of the colon taken above the line of demarcation will confirm this normal color.

The goal of treatment is the reduction of symptoms. Since these tend to come and go, and the hazards of ulcerative proctitis are low, medication usually is given only for short periods of time. For the patient with ulcerative proctitis, neither the disease nor the treatment is likely to cause major problems. However, there are some patients who continue to have active disease in this small segment of bowel, despite medications.

CROHN'S DISEASE

In 1932, Drs. Crohn, Leon Ginzburg, and Gordon D. Oppenheimer of the Mount Sinai Hospital in New York first described a disease of the ileum, or last segment of small intestine, which they distinguished from intestinal tuberculosis. The disease they described was characterized by insidious onset, weakness, fever, and nonbloody diarrhea. Because it appeared to affect only the terminal or end part of the ileum, they called the disease terminal ileitis or regional ileitis to indicate that only a portion of the intestine was involved. The choice of the term *terminal ileitis* was unfortunate, since some patients mistakenly thought that their disease was terminal or fatal, which it generally is not.

The disease as described by Crohn, Ginzburg, and Oppenheimer produces a marked thickening of the intestinal wall causing a narrowing of the bowel channel (lumen). In extreme cases, the narrowing is so severe that it prevents the passage of intestinal contents and causes obstruction. In other cases the inflammation spreads beyond the confines of the bowel wall and penetrates to adjacent loops of bowel, to other organs such as the bladder, or to the skin surface. These abnormal connections are called fistulas (fistulae). Under the microscope, distinguishing features of Crohn's disease are the involvement of the entire thickness of bowel wall, and the presence of granulomas. (A granuloma is a microscopic lesion caused by the migration of inflammatory cells to an area. Granulomas are seen in 30 to 50 percent of cases of Crohn's disease, but never in ulcerative colitis.

As time passed it became evident that the same pathological process which inflames the terminal ileum could also affect any part of the digestive tract, such as the esophagus, stomach, duodenum, jejunum, and colon, either alone or in combination. At first these inflammations were thought to be separate diseases, but when granulomas were found in these cases as well, it was evident that this disease—Crohn's disease—could involve any segment of the gastrointestinal tract from the mouth to the anus. There is still a good deal of confusion about terminology in Crohn's disease. Despite the persistence of older terms like ileitis, regional enteritis, and granulomatous colitis, the almost universal use today of the name Crohn's disease means that this is now considered as one disease no matter where it appears.

In most areas of the world where it is found, Crohn's ileocolitis (involving both ileum and colon) is the most common form of the disease, followed by Crohn's disease confined to the ileum. Together, these two distributions account for at least 80 percent of all cases of Crohn's disease. Crohn's disease of the colon alone is seen in about 15 percent of all cases and can be mistaken for chronic ulcerative colitis. There are several important features that distinguish the two diseases. In Crohn's colitis, the rectum frequently is normal and there may be asymmetrical "skip areas" in the colon (contiguous areas of diseased and healthy bowel). In chronic ulcerative colitis, the rectum is almost always involved, and the inflammation in the colon is uniform and continuous.

Extraintestinal or systemic involvement is common in Crohn's disease as in chronic ulcerative colitis, but the presence of a fistula makes the diagnosis of Crohn's disease much more likely. This is especially true when there is a recto-vaginal fistula (an abnormal connection between the rectum and vagina), which may occur in both diseases. A description of the complications of both Crohn's disease and ulcerative colitis will be found in Chapter 5.

It is extremely unfortunate that a correct diagnosis of Crohn's disease may not be reached for months or even years. This tendency to late diagnosis in Crohn's disease results from its slow, insidious onset (usually without a dramatic precipitating event), its vague symptoms resembling those of other diseases, and a lack of knowledge about the disease among many physicians. Unfortunately, symptoms of Crohn's disease are often thought (incorrectly) to arise from emotional causes, and some patients are treated mistakenly with tranquilizers or psychotherapy while symptoms persist until a proper diagnosis is finally made.

The diagnosis of Crohn's disease begins with a careful history and a complete physical examination. A history suggestive of Crohn's disease includes weight loss, fever, abdominal pain, and diarrhea that often awakens the patient at night. It is always important to tell the physician if any other members of the family are known to have either ulcerative colitis or Crohn's disease. Studies have shown that 15 to 30 percent of patients have another close family member or a distant relative with one or the other disease. A detailed history and thorough physical examination should alert a careful physican to order appropriate studies, including blood tests (for anemia and evidence of inflammation), stool examinations, barium X-ray studies (barium enema, upper GI series, and small bowel X-ray examination), sigmoidoscopy, biopsy, and, when indicated, colonoscopy. These tests will be covered in detail in Chapter 4.

As in ulcerative colitis, malignant tumors of the intestinal tract have been found in Crohn's disease of the colon, and, extremely rarely, in Crohn's disease of the ileum; but their incidence is far lower than in ulcerative colitis. This subject, as well as the medical and surgical treatment of Crohn's disease, will be covered in subsequent chapters.

2

WHO GETS CROHN'S DISEASE AND ULCERATIVE COLITIS?

Who gets Crohn's disease and ulcerative colitis? Are more men than women afflicted? How old are most patients? Where else in the world do people suffer from these illnesses?

These challenging questions are tackled by the branch of research medicine known as epidemiology. Epidemiologists study the distribution of disease in human populations. But they do far more than count cases of disease. By searching out details such as age, sex, race, place of residence, diet, or occupation of patients, epidemiologists are able to uncover "risk factors" common to groups of patients with the same disease.

This kind of "backward look" at people who have already been diagnosed with an illness is called a retrospective study. It is often the first step in identifying which among a large number of factors might be responsible for causing a disease. A well-known example of this method of study was the discovery of cigarette smoking as a risk factor in lung cancer. Study after study piled up evidence that people who developed lung cancer were also likely to be cigarette smokers. In another example, retrospective studies showed that women in their middle years who developed strokes or blood clots in the leg had a history of having used oral contraceptives. In both examples, epidemiologic studies provided the first clues.

The search for risk factors in IBD has been marked by a good deal of frustration. Epidemiologists begin by finding all the diagnosed cases of Crohn's disease or ulcerative colitis in what is called a "defined population." A defined population is one that is somewhat geographically self-contained—an island is an extreme example—and where people do not generally go outside the area to obtain health care. The epidemiologist searches hospital, physician, and clinic records for all diagnosed cases of Crohn's disease and ulcerative colitis, and calculates rates of occurrence of these diseases in the population. This is difficult to do in the United States, where few defined populations exist and where the records of private physicians are not generally available to the epidemiologist. Nevertheless, we do know a good deal about the distribution of IBD in the United States from studies that have been done, enough to be able to answer these important questions about who gets IBD.

HOW MANY PEOPLE IN THE UNITED STATES HAVE IBD?

Since we can count only those cases of IBD discharged from hospitals in the United States, and not those that are treated out of the hospital by private physicians, the data that we have will tend to underestimate the problem. About 30,000 new cases of IBD are admitted to U.S. hospitals each year. There are at least 500,000 people who suffer chronically from IBD (slightly more from ulcerative colitis than Crohn's disease), according to hospital discharge diagnoses in the United States. But considering the delay in diagnosis of Crohn's disease (approximately three to five years) and the fact that many people are not hospitalized for their disease, this figure could easily be 1 or 2 million.

Epidemiologists tell us that the occurrence of ulcerative colitis has remained steady over the last few decades, and may be decreasing through the 1980s. Occurrence of Crohn's disease, on the other hand, has been increasing steadily over the past decade, so that its rate of occurrence is about the same as ulcerative colitis. However, recent studies in the United States, England, Scotland, and Sweden predict that this rapid increase will level off during the 1980s.

IN WHICH PARTS OF THE WORLD CAN IBD BE FOUND?

IBD is predominantly a disease of the developed world. The countries reporting the highest occurrence rates of both Crohn's disease and ulcerative colitis are the United States, England, Scotland, the Scandinavian countries, a few countries in Western and Central Europe, and Israel. The risk of developing either disease is about five times greater among Jews living in the United States and Europe, although in the Jewish population of Israel, rates have not been very high. When the disease is seen among Jews in Israel, it is predominantly in those of European or American background (*Ashkenazim*) and not among Jews from Middle Eastern countries (*Sephardim*). A long-term analysis of IBD in these two groups may reveal the significance of environmental factors on these diseases.

IBD has generally not been found among peoples living in Asia (except Japan), equatorial Africa, and South

14

America, areas that have poor sanitation, lower nutritional standards, poor food storage facilities, and a high frequency of diarrheal diseases caused by bacteria and parasites. Epidemiologists have observed an inverse relationship between the frequency of these infectious diarrheas (a marker of the underdeveloped world) and the frequency of IBD. In other words, the higher the standard of living, the greater the prevalence of IBD. Epidemiologists feel that poor access to health care alone could not account for this difference.

COULD DIET EXPLAIN THE DIFFERENCES?

IBD is common among those people who eat a "Western" diet, one high in animal protein and fat, with much smaller quantities of vegetables, fruits, and cereal grains than are consumed in non-Western diets. Over the past century, people in the developed world have increased their intake of refined sugars, kept their intake of saturated fat high, and have used salt liberally.

However, studies within the Western world have not found that those persons who suffer from IBD differ in their food intake from those who do not have IBD. In other words, the mere fact of eating this diet, which has produced great longevity and generally good health for the entire population does not seem to induce IBD in more than a very small fraction of the population.

WHAT ABOUT ENVIRONMENTAL FACTORS?

So far, epidemiologists have found no specific risk for IBD among rural or urban dwellers in Western populations. No specific occupation has large numbers of IBD sufferers, and no environmental contaminant has been found to cause clusters of cases in certain geographic areas. The slight predominanace of IBD in urban over rural areas can be explaned in other ways, including the availability of better medical facilities for making diagnoses. As poorer segments of Western society have more access to medical care, IBD is being found among them in proportions not very different from those of their more educated and affluent neighbors.

IS RACE A FACTOR IN DEVELOPING IBD?

Although IBD occurs rarely among Orientals, Asiatic Indians, American Indians, and Africans, when these groups migrate to Western societies they do develop IBD, although the numbers and frequencies are still lower than among Caucasians. Among United States blacks there has been a rather rapidly increasing prevalence of both ulcerative colitis and Crohn's disease. In studies done in the late 1970s, the rate of occurrence of these diseases in black women aged 20 to 40 was almost identical with that of white women of the same age. Some have thought this might reflect the widespread use of oral contraceptives in the period between 1965 and 1975, but whether these women actually used such medications is not known. Among U.S. black men, the frequency of IBD is definitely lower than among white males, and it is still unusual, but not rare, to find American black families with more than one IBD sufferer. Among blacks who do get IBD, the disease does not seem any less severe than among whites.

AT WHAT AGE DOES IBD GENERALLY BEGIN?

Most large Western populations of IBD patients show two definite peaks in age of onset. Although IBD can begin at any age, there is a concentration of cases beginning about age 12 and accelerating through age 28, then tapering down to a very low incidence of new cases at about age 40 to 50. After age 50 there is a smaller second wave of new cases, which continues for about a decade. This second wave is of great interest. Does it represent a new group of persons who have become at risk for the disease, or are these people suffering from a different disease that only looks like IBD? To what extent does the aging process itself contribute to this new wave of cases? We cannot provide definitive answers to any of these questions but must await better tools for their investigation.

IS IBD A GENETIC DISEASE?

Most disorders that are acquired after childhood represent the interplay of environmental elements and genetic factors, and are inherited in an undetermined fashion. We do know that Crohn's disease and ulcerative colitis tend to run in families. Children having a parent with IBD are more likely to have inherited some of those genes probably necessary for developing these diseases, and are more likely to have IBD than the general population. Studies have shown that between 15 and 30 percent of patients have a relative with either disease. But there does not seem to be any clear-cut pattern to the appearance of the diseases, even when they cluster in families.

Since research has not yet been able to associate these diseases with specific genes that govern their transmission, IBD is considered to be "familial," and not "genetic" in the strict sense of the word.

Given the absence of typical patterns of distribution in the family, there have been no probability studies on whether the disease will affect a predicted number of children or skip a generation. In other words, the laws of Mendelian inheritance as we know them do not seem to apply to these illnesses.

More importantly, physicians are very reluctant to discourage a couple from having a child because of any likelihood that the child might "inherit" a form of IBD. There is simply not enough known to be able to counsel parents on this factor. Furthermore, Crohn's disease and ulcerative colitis could appear in mild form, if at all, and are certainly not considered terminal illnesses. So genetic counseling is not practiced with IBD.

We will probably learn a great deal more about the possible genetic aspects of Crohn's disease and ulcerative colitis from intensive studies of families in which more than one member has the disease. The feasibility of such studies is now being considered by NFIC.

3

WHAT CAUSES CROHN'S DISEASE AND ULCERATIVE COLITIS?

For many years both Crohn's disease and ulcerative colitis were confused with various infections involving the bowel. Even today, the occurrence of IBD may be "rare" in tropical countries because of the difficulty in differentiating it from the frequent intestinal infections that occur in these populations. For example, it took a long time to distinguish Crohn's disease from tuberculosis. Many years before the description of ileitis, pathologists often lamented the fact that they had seen what appeared to be tuberculosis of the intestine, but no tuberculosis organisms could be found. These early cases were undoubtedly Crohn's disease. Ulcerative colitis, likewise, has often been confused with amebiasis and salmonella infection and, more recently, with campylobacter infections.

In recent years, an imbalance between the astronomical numbers and types of intestinal bacteria that live within the colon has been implicated in these diseases. In fact, there has been much recent interest in an organism called *Clos-*

19

tridium difficile. As mentioned in Chapter 1, this bacterium is occasionally found in people taking certain antibiotics, and can be the cause of diarrhea and colon inflammation. The antibiotics apparently kill some of the "good" intestinal bacteria which in turn help keep the clostridia in check. With the use of antibiotics, the "good" organisms are eliminated and the "bad" organisms can now grow and produce a toxic colitis. At present, some investigators feel that this may account for some flare-ups in ulcerative colitis. However, other studies have failed to show that the use of antibiotics is a trigger.

THE SEARCH FOR A VIRAL AGENT

Viruses have been examined as possible causative agents in both Crohn's disease and ulcerative colitis. The best way to test for viruses is to try to detect their antibodies in the patient's blood. Antibodies are protective substances produced by some white blood cells (lymphocytes), which react with and help destroy viruses. One possible correlation has been found by isolating an antibody to the cytomegalic inclusion virus (CMV) seen only in the blood of ulcerative colitis patients. However, at the present time it is thought that this virus is a secondary invader that attacks the weakened intestinal lining, and not a primary cause of the disease.

Viruses have also been sought by the inoculation of Crohn's disease and ulcerative colitis material into embryonic eggs, suckling mice, guinea pigs, miniature swine, rabbits, and a broad variety of tissue culture lines (Figure 2). Until 1970 these approaches had gone unrewarded. Then Drs. D. N. Mitchell and R. J. Rees reported that by injecting Crohn's disease tissue into footpads of mice, they could produce microscopic changes that resembled those seen in

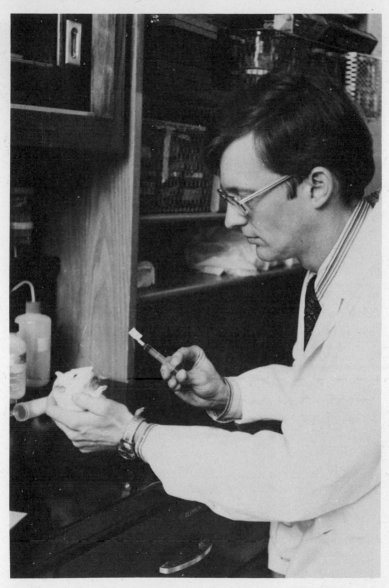

Figure 2. Research sponsored by the National Foundation for Ileitis & Colitis is investigating the way in which certain bacteria or viruses might alter the body's immune system, its natural protection against disease.

Crohn's disease. Unfortunately, these findings were not confirmed by other investigators. It now appears that in an effort to remove possible contaminating bacteria from the Crohn's disease tissue, the investigators had passed the material through filters with pores large enough to allow viruses to pass through but small enough to trap and exclude the larger bacteria. Some fibers from the filter, acting as a foreign body, probably produced these microscopic changes.

Recently, attempts to grow infectious agents from Crohn's tissue culture have been pursued. In 1975, Dr. M. D. Aronson reported that inoculation of Crohn's disease tissue into certain types of tissue cultures could produce a "cytopathic effect." This "cytopathic effect" means that there were changes in the tissue culture cells that were not found in the uninoculated cells. This "effect" could be passed onto other tissue cultures. These findings were confirmed by Dr. Gary Gitnick and his collaborators; further studies suggest, however, that the "cytopathic" agent is not a living organism but perhaps some type of toxic protein or chemical.

BACTERIA UNDER SUSPICION

Currently, considerable research is being carried out to identify other possible causative organisms. Interest centers around the role of anaerobic bacteria—bacteria that cannot tolerate oxygen. The drug metronidazole (Flagyl), which is very effective against anaerobic bacteria, has been shown to reduce the inflammation of perianal (surrounding the anus) fistulas and abscesses that sometimes complicate Crohn's disease. Some recent studies from Holland indicate that two special types of anaerobes are found in increased numbers in patients with Crohn's disease. Interestingly, antibodies to these agents were found in a significant percentage of patients with Crohn's disease, but not in patients with ulcerative colitis.

Mycobacteria are another group of organisms that have been studied extensively as possible perpetrators of IBD. Not only has Crohn's disease been confused with tuberculosis, which is caused by *Mycobacterium tuberculosis,* but it also bears many similarities to a mycobacterium-caused illness found in animals. In addition, an effective drug in the treatment of tuberculosis, paraminosalicylic acid, is closely related to 5-aminosalicylic acid, the effective component of sulfasalazine (Azulfidine), a drug frequently prescribed for IBD. In 1978, Dr. Burnham, using a special type of culture medium, isolated a cell-wall-defective bacterium that he thought was a *Mycobacterium kansasi.* More studies of this interesting agent are awaited.

The prolonged inability of scientists to find a specific virus or bacterium as the cause of IBD suggests that there may be many organisms individually able to initiate the disease, or that there may be an interaction of multiple agents, no one of which by itself could produce IBD.

THE IMMUNE RESPONSE IN IBD

A second area of great interest is the search for a possible abnormal immune response in individuals with IBD. Many researchers feel that the diseases might result when the body's defenses respond abnormally to an infectious or toxic agent. One possibility is that an abnormality *decreases* the immune response so that a developing infection cannot be controlled by the body, resulting in IBD. Another theory is that an abnormality creates an *excessive* immune response so that innocent bystander cells, such as those lining the intestine, are destroyed together with the offending agent.

To understand a little more about immunological mechanisms in IBD, it is helpful to review the basics of immunology. There are three types of white cells that help us in our resistance to infections. These cells are the monocytes, the polymorphonuclear leukocytes ("polys"), and the lymphocytes. We will not discuss the first two types of cells, because our knowledge of them relative to IBD is at present very limited. However, what is known suggests that in IBD patients there may be crucial changes in these cells as well.

THREE TYPES OF LYMPHOCYTES

Lymphocytes, on the other hand, have been studied rather extensively. A lymphocyte is "born" in the bone marrow. From here, some of these cells migrate to a gland in the neck called the thymus. There they mature into T-cells, whereupon they assume one of at least three types of functions. They can become 1) cytotoxic cells, which destroy invading organisms or other abnormal cells, such as cancer cells, 2) helper cells, which help the B-cell (see below) to make antibodies, or 3) suppressor cells, which help hold down an immune response so that it does not become excessive. There are, therefore, considerable checks and balances on the immune response by the interaction of these cells when they are functioning properly.

Other cells from the bone marrow go to the lymph nodes and spleen and are called B-cells. These cells mature and with the help of the T-cells become antibody-producing cells or plasma cells. An antibody is a specific protein molecule made by the plasma cell that reacts with an "antigen," usually some foreign substance with which the body tissues come into contact. The antibody usually binds to the antigen, which, in turn, leads to the antigen's destruction.

A third type of lymphocyte, called the K-cell, is not really well characterized, but appears to be responsible for antibody-dependent cell cytotoxicity, or destruction.

ANTICOLON ANTIBODIES

In 1959, Drs. O. Broberger and P. Perlmann described anticolon (i.e., specific for the colon) antibodies in the blood of patients with ulcerative colitis. Similar antibodies were later identified in the blood of patients with Crohn's disease. The antibodies reacted not only against colon cells but also against certain intestinal bacteria. It was thought that these bacteria, of the *Escherichia coli* family (a group of largely harmless bacteria found in the human intestine), and the colon shared a common antigen. It was theorized that perhaps an infection with these bacteria led to the development of an antibody that could not recognize the difference between the bacteria and the colon. The antibody presumably reacted against the colon and produced colitis. Unfortunately for this hypothesis, Drs. Broberger and Perlmann found that these antibodies did not cause cell damage when they were added to intestinal colon cells in tissue culture. However, they were able to show that the white blood cells of patients with either ulcerative colitis or Crohn's disease were capable of causing cell destruction when these cells were added to the colon cells growing in tissue culture. This work was confirmed and amplified by the work of Dr. Roy G. Shorter at the Mayo Clinic, who also found that normal lymphocytes could be made to react against the colon tissue cells if they were first incubated in the sera (the fluid portion of the blood) of patients with IBD. Further studies by Broberger and Perlmann suggested that this was an antibody-dependent cell cytotoxicity type of reaction that required the K-cell for the colon cell destruction. However, recent investigators have actually isolated lymphocytes from the small and large intestines of patients with either IBD or cancer and have found that there is a virtual absence of K-cells in these tissues. Nevertheless, there is still considerable interest in the role of the K-cell in the damage seen in IBD, with the hope that further experimental work will lead to clarification of these findings.

ANTIGEN-ANTIBODY COMPLEXES IN IBD

When an antibody attaches itself to an antigen circulating in the blood, an antigen-antibody complex is formed. These complexes can cause damage when they are deposited in tissues. Certain factors released by these trapped complexes cause the migration of white blood cells and other blood components into the area where they produce tissue damage. Colitis can be produced experimentally in rabbits if antigen-antibody complexes are infused into the blood of these animals while, at the same time, the colon is slightly irritated. This irritation of the colon causes the complexes to be deposited in the inflamed area, thus producing a severe colitis. Many investigators have found these complexes in the blood of patients with IBD. However, their exact role relative to IBD is at the present time unclear. Skin rashes, arthritis, and eye inflammation are found frequently in IBD and in other diseases, such as lupus erythematosus, where these complexes are also known to circulate.

How can we put all this complex information together? This chapter has considered both the search for infectious agents and the investigation of an abnormal immune response in IBD. This does not mean that these are actually separate and distinct approaches. In fact, the two approaches probably complement one another. Some investigators feel that the immunologic changes occur after the

IBD has started. If ulcerative colitis and/or Crohn's disease prove to be caused by an infectious agent, there still must be a discrepancy in the immune response that permits one person to overcome the infection while another endures a chronic, often unrelenting disease. A similar situation is seen in people who become infected with hepatitis B virus. Some get over the hepatitis completely; others develop a chronic infection; others live with the virus with no damage to the liver, and some develop cancer. Even if these diseases are truly what we call "autoimmune," they perhaps still need some type of infectious agent to initiate the process.

At this stage in our search for the cause of IBD, both infectious agents and the abnormal immune response continue to offer the most promising leads. As we begin to understand more about the ability of the normal intestine to respond to infection, we will gain more insight into what goes wrong in these illnesses.

4

DIAGNOSING CROHN'S DISEASE AND ULCERATIVE COLITIS

THE MEDICAL HISTORY

Since Crohn's disease and ulcerative colitis may first appear in many different guises, it is important that the physician take a careful medical history. Often, the patient's description of the symptoms together with the physical examination will be enough to arrive at a diagnosis of IBD.

An individual with either disease may become severely ill over a short period of time—days, or even hours—or the symptoms can appear so slowly that neither physician nor patient suspects the diagnosis for months, or even years. These patients may have a history of intermittent diarrhea and abdominal pain that no physician felt was significant. It is not unusual for persons with Crohn's disease first to undergo surgery for removal of the appendix before the surgeon reaches the correct diagnosis. There are other individuals whose only symptoms are fatigue, low-grade fever, and loss of weight.

THREE CLASSIC DIAGNOSTIC SIGNS

Generally, most people with IBD experience three major symptoms: diarrhea, abdominal pain, and fever. The diarrhea may be mild, moderate, or quite severe. The nature of the diarrhea is always an important clue for the physician suspecting IBD and often helps him or her to localize the area of the bowel involvement. What is most important to observe is whether there is a nocturnal pattern, i.e., does the patient awaken during the night with an urge to move the bowels. Nocturnal diarrhea strongly suggests that there is organic disease such as IBD, and *not* a functional problem such as the irritable bowel syndrome (IBS). In Crohn's disease, the diarrhea is usually not bloody, although bleeding can occur if the left side of the colon is diseased. In ulcerative colitis the diarrhea is almost always bloody, and may contain mucus and pus as well.

The type of abdominal pain felt by the patient may also vary depending on the severity and the location of bowel inflammation. In ulcerative colitis, the pain is usually crampy in nature and is often relieved after a bowel movement. In Crohn's disease, pain is generally more persistent and may be aggravated by eating, especially if there is narrowing of the intestine. Nausea, sometimes with vomiting, may accompany the pain. Perianal abscess, fissure, or fistula may cause severe pain.

Fever in IBD may be low-grade (100°–101° F) or may run as high as 103°–104° F when the disease is severe or when an abscess is present. In either case, fever is always an important sign. Persons running low-grade temperatures may not be aware of it, and may show an irritability or lethargy that is annoying to friends and family. In some patients, fever may break during the night, causing profuse perspiration. To the alert physician, these "night sweats" are a significant clue to the seriousness of the illness.

OTHER IMPORTANT CLUES

There are many signs suggesting Crohn's disease or ulcerative colitis in people who have none of the classic symptoms mentioned above. Sores inside the mouth (aphthous ulcers) often occur in Crohn's disease. Clubbing (prominence) of the fingernails, reddening of the eyes, joint pains, skin lesions, and growth impairment in children are all important signs of IBD that can occur *before* there is any disturbance in bowel activity at all. (See Chapter 5 for a complete description of the systemic (nonintestinal) manifestations of inflammatory bowel disease.) The presence of any of these signs should alert the physician to consider IBD and to proceed with diagnostic studies of the bowel.

Other manifestations in the anal region deserve special mention. Perianal symptoms (pain, abnormal drainage of mucus and pus, or abscesses around the anus) occur very frequently in Crohn's disease, often months or years before bowel symptoms occur. The presence of a perianal fistula (abnormal channel draining from bowel to anal area) in a person who is experiencing diarrhea, fever, and weight loss, or even the presence of an anal skin tab, with no other symptoms, strongly suggests that bowel studies should be done to rule out Crohn's disease. Surgery should *not* be performed on the anus or rectum until the diagnostic evaluation is complete.

Since early diagnosis and prompt, adequate treatment of Crohn's disease and ulcerative colitis can help control the symptoms of both diseases, it is very important to report early symptoms to your physician. If he or she is unable to evaluate or treat these symptoms, your doctor should refer you to a gastroenterologist, a specialist in the diagnosis and treatment of digestive diseases.

THE PHYSICAL EXAMINATION

After taking a careful medical history of your symptoms, your physician will perform a thorough physical examination. He or she may find, besides weight loss, low-grade fever, and pallor from anemia, abdominal tenderness in the right lower quadrant of the abdomen in ileitis, or, in either ulcerative colitis or Crohn's disease, in areas overlying the colon. In Crohn's disease of the ileum, there may be a tender abdominal mass in the lower abdomen on the right side caused by a thickened, inflamed ileum. Examination of the perianal area may reveal a variety of abnormalities including hemorrhoids, an anal fissure (a painful crack in the lining of the anus), perianal abscess or a painless anal skin tab. In Crohn's disease, the inflammatory response in the anal area may be very complex. Several false openings called sinus tracts may discharge purulent or fecal material. In addition, there may be thickened tender mounds of tissue around the anus resembling portions of a cauliflower. In women, there may be a fistula between the rectum and the vagina.

Rectal examination in ulcerative colitis may reveal nothing abnormal, but occasionally there is subtle irregularity of tissue indicating ulceration of the lining. Blood from the lining may appear on the glove of the physician's examining finger. In Crohn's disease, there may be severe narrowing of the rectal segment in the form of an extensive stricture through which the physician's finger cannot pass.

In examining a child or teenager suspected of having IBD, the physician should measure the important parameters of growth such as height, weight, and evidence of sexual maturation. These are covered in detail in Chapter 10.

LABORATORY TESTS

No specific laboratory test nor combination of them will yield a definitive diagnosis of Crohn's disease or ulcerative colitis. The results of laboratory tests must be correlated with clinical and X-ray findings before a diagnosis can be made. The white blood cell count (WBC) and erythrocyte (red blood cell) sedimentation rate (ESR) may be elevated, confirming an inflammatory process somewhere in the body. The stool examination may be positive for hidden (occult) blood. Hemoglobin and hematocrit (the ratio of red blood cells to whole blood) may be lower than normal, indicating anemia. There may be many causes for this anemia, including a deficiency of iron (as a result of the passage of blood into the stool), a deficiency in vitamin B-12 caused by poor absorption of this vitamin from the ileum in Crohn's disease, or folic acid deficiency caused by inflammation in the upper small intestine (jejunum) or by sulfasalazine, if this drug has been used. A wide variety of other laboratory tests may be helpful in diagnosing the disease, including liver function tests to determine whether the liver has been affected, and tests measuring the absorption of nutrients. Low serum albumin (one of the proteins circulating in the blood) is a reasonably accurate indication that the patient's overall protein stores may be depleted.

DIAGNOSTIC PROCEDURES FOR IBD

In the further evaluation of a patient with diarrhea, a sigmoidoscopy followed by a barium X ray of the colon is a logical starting point. However, in most cases it is first necessary to examine the stools carefully for other causes of diarrhea and inflammation such as ova and parasites (giardia and ameba), harmful bacteria (such as shigella, salmonella, campylobacter, and yersinia), and clostridia toxin (found in a type of colitis caused by the use of antibiotics). Both sigmoidoscopy and stool examinations must be done prior to the barium enema study because once barium has been instilled into the colon, the rectum and sigmoid are coated white for many days, making it impossible to inspect this area carefully, and very difficult to identify these organisms.

Sigmoidoscopy is a test in which a fiberoptic tube with a light at one end is passed through the anus to inspect the rectum and the sigmoid colon. The physician looks through the viewing end and can see the lining quite clearly. The test can be done quickly in the doctor's office without too much discomfort. Sedation is not generally needed.

The sigmoidoscopy should precede a barium enema X ray. At the time of sigmoidoscopy, the physician may decide to take a small specimen (biopsy) from the colon and rectum for examination under the microscope. This biopsy is almost always painless, and may be of help in distinguishing Crohn's disease from ulcerative colitis.

If a patient is acutely ill and the sigmoidoscopy reveals changes characteristic of inflammatory bowel disease, the X ray of the colon should be postponed. Later, when the patient's condition has stabilized, the barium enema can be performed to confirm the diagnosis and to delineate the extent of disease. On the other hand, if the sigmoidoscopic examination is negative, the physician may decide to perform the barium enema on the same day in an effort to obtain as much information as possible to make a proper diagnosis.

PREPARING FOR X-RAY EXAMINATION

The Barium Enema

Most radiologists have a standard set of instructions for patients who are about to undergo barium enema examination. Usually a strong purge is ordered to remove residual stool that would otherwise show up on the X ray. However, in persons suspected of having colitis, it is unnecessary to purge the colon since most of the stool has already been eliminated as diarrhea. In fact, the use of harsh substances such as castor oil or soapsuds enemas may cause a flare-up of underlying colitis. With this in mind, the standard instructions for bowel preparation should be adapted to the condition of the patient. The choices for preparing the IBD patient for X ray are the following:

1. If the patient is quite ill and is experiencing severe abdominal pain and fever, no preparation should be administered and a sigmoidoscopy alone should be done. An X-ray film of the abdomen *without barium* can be taken to try to find any abnormality in the rest of the colon.

2. If the patient is not seriously ill but is having diarrhea, a sigmoidoscopy and barium enema can be done with little or no preparation. For minimal preparation, a gentle tap water enema (1 quart) may be given one to two hours prior to the sigmoidoscopy and barium enema. If there is severe abdominal pain as the tap water is being slowly instilled, even this mild preparation should be discontinued.

3. If the patient is having diarrhea mixed with semisolid stools, he or she can be given one-half bottle of citrate of magnesia the afternoon before the X ray, and clear liquids for 24 hours prior to the X ray. The patient can then be evaluated on the morning of the X ray. A tap water enema (1 quart) one to two hours prior to the barium enema may be given.

Taking a Tap Water Enema

Water for this enema should be warm (about body temperature) and should be introduced while the patient is lying on the left side. The tip of the syringe or tubing should be lubricated with petroleum jelly to avoid irritating the anus.

Care should be taken to avoid introducing air into the colon, which will cause discomfort and the need to evacuate. After about one-third to one-half quart of water has been administered, the patient should roll over to the *right* side and finish taking the enema. This helps distribute the water evenly in the colon. Water should be held in the colon as long as possible before evacuating (2 to 5 minutes, if possible).

It is especially important for the patient to observe the waste that is expelled before flushing the toilet. If it becomes excessively bloody, he or she should stop the preparation at once and alert the physician. If the fluid is not bloody and appears thin and pale brown in color, the preparation is complete and no additional enemas are needed. This point is emphasized because some physicians often give instructions that tap water enemas be taken on the morning of the examination "until clear." The patient then supposes that the water on evacuation from the colon must be very clean, an impossibility.

When the patient is hospitalized, it is especially important for the physician to tell the patient directly which preparation is to be used. This will enable the patient to avoid any possible nursing error in which castor oil (a routine cathartic for most barium enemas) might be used by mistake. The patient should also know exactly what type of enema is planned, and should refuse any preparation containing soapsuds.

If the inflammation of the rectum is significant, and especially if there is a stricture (narrowing) of the rectum, only a soft rubber tube should ever be used in the rectum. The general practice of many radiologists is to insert a tube and then inflate a balloon in this tube to a diameter that occludes the rectal opening and prevents the leaking of barium. Inflating a balloon in an actively diseased or narrowed rectum could be harmful, and since most rectal disease is diagnosed by sigmoidoscopy, before the barium series is done, it is important that the patient and physician know the extent of the disease and insist that the rectum be treated with care.

Although it is usual practice following a barium enema to administer oral or rectal medications to encourage the removal of residual barium from the colon, this procedure is generally not followed if a person is found to have colitis.

UPPER GASTROINTESTINAL (GI) SERIES WITH SMALL BOWEL EXAMINATION

When a GI series with small bowel follow-through is performed, there is no bowel preparation at all. The patient should simply eat nothing after midnight the night before. On the morning of the X ray, he or she will drink a measured amount of liquid barium, a thick, chalky substance obtainable in several flavors. The patient should generally expect to spend two to four hours in the X-ray department, during which time barium flows through the small intestine until it finally enters the terminal ileum and proximal portion of the colon. At this point, if Crohn's disease of the ileum is suspected, the radiologist will generally take additional X rays of this segment, frequently using a special compression paddle to separate adjoining barium-filled loops so that the last loop of ileum can be seen clearly. Radiologic changes of the ileum that are characteristic of Crohn's disease of the ileum include narrowing of the intestinal passage (lumen), distortion of the lining so that the normal pattern is lost, and the presence of linear wisps of barium that sometimes form a cross-hatched appearance.

An X-ray examination of the colon may reveal a flattening of the normally rounded symmetric convolutions of the colon (haustrations). Tiny ulcerations may be visible, and the colon is frequently in spasm. In ulcerative colitis of many years' duration, there may occasionally be strictures. The radiologist also looks carefully for malignant tumors of the colon, especially if the disease involves most or all of the colon and has been present more than seven to ten years. An increased frequency of colon and rectal cancer in long-standing ulcerative colitis makes close surveillance advisable. Chapter 9 contains a detailed explanation of the risk of cancer in IBD and describes methods for surveillance.

COLONOSCOPY

In some cases of inflammatory bowel disease, the precise diagnosis may still be in doubt, even after careful history and physical examination, laboratory tests, and X rays. In these instances, the technique of flexible fiberoptic endoscopy may be of great benefit in distinguishing whether a patient has ulcerative colitis or Crohn's disease.

The flexible colonoscope, an endoscope first developed in the 1960s, provides a direct view of the inner lining of the colon. Light is directed into the intestinal tract from outside the patient by bundles of tiny glass light-carrying rods within the colonoscope. A single lens at the end of the instrument focuses the view inside the intestinal tract on the pinhead-sized bundle of glass fibers, and a strong magnifying lens near the observer's eye enlarges the image to a picture ten times greater than life-size. Still pictures, movies, and videotapes can be made through the use of a camera mounted on the observer eyepiece device (Figure 3).

The new fiberoptic scope is about as flexible as a garden hose and can be tied into a knot while still transmitting an accurate image through its entire length. The instrument is advanced gently through the rectum and along the colon in

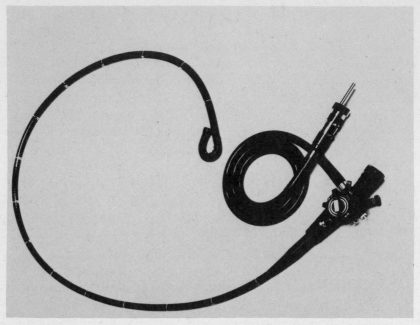

Figure 3. The fiberoptic colonoscope.

a guided, carefully controlled manner. As the physician manipulates the dial controls to direct the tip through the intestinal tract, the colonoscope can show directly every portion of the large intestine.

A small tube runs the entire length of the instrument, through which a biopsy forceps can be passed. The forceps have a small "mouth" that can be opened and closed by the endoscopist or an assistant. When the forceps jaws are opened and advanced to contact the lining of the colon, they "bite off" a tiny fragment of tissue that is sent to the pathology laboratory for microscopic diagnosis. The taking of such a biopsy specimen is not painful, since the large intestine has no pain fibers. A suction machine can be attached to this tubelike channel to suction out fluid from the intestinal tract, and a small "windshield wiper" system at the intestinal end cleans mucus and fluid from the observing lens. The physician has a control that permits insertion of air into the colon to distend the bowel and improve visibility. The tip of the flexible instrument can be bent in a sharp arc by dial controls attached to directional guide wires at the head portion of the instrument. The entire fiberoptic instrument is about the width of an index finger and is truly one of the marvels of medical instrumentation.

Risks and Rewards

Although the fiberoptic colonoscope has revolutionized the approach to diseases of the intestinal tract, it is not intended for use in every patient with intestinal problems. In spite of its capability of showing pathology directly and obtaining biopsy specimens simultaneously, the instrument has certain drawbacks. The intestinal tract is not straight; loops of bowel curve and wind back and forth, so that the configuration of the colon in the abdomen is more like a pretzel than a horseshoe. Manipulating a six-foot-long instrument around all of the various bends of the colon takes considerable skill. There is a possibility that the colon-oscope might perforate the bowel wall. This is a rare oc-currence but is the most serious complication of endoscopy and is usually treated by emergency surgery. In a patient with an inflammatory condition of the large intestine, where there is an alteration in the integrity of the colon wall, perforation is a greater risk. Consequently, it is essential that a colonoscopy be performed only by physicians skilled in the use of the instrument, and *only* when the information to be derived from colonoscopy is of great benefit—such as in the search for malignant changes, or in the formulation of an important change in therapeutic approach.

The patient advised to have a colonoscopy or other endoscopic procedure should ask the physician:
1. Why is the procedure being done?
2. What information will be learned that could not be learned using other tests?

3. How will the results of the procedure alter the physician's management of the disease?

Preparing for a Colonoscopy

Once the physician has decided to perform a colonoscopy, the lining of the intestine must be clean and devoid of solid fecal material to permit full viewing of the bowel wall. In the patient with a normal colon, a liquid diet is necessary for a minimum of twenty-four hours before the exam, followed by a castor oil purge. Residual fecal contents are then evacuated with the aid of cleansing enemas. Such a vigorous "prep" should not be used in the patient with inflammatory bowel disease. There is a possiblility that the use of laxatives may cause a flare-up of the disease. For a patient with inflammatory bowel disease who is undergoing colonoscopy, a liquid diet for forty-eight hours before the exam is suggested. During the first twenty-four hours the patient may have full liquids (including any variety of soup, milk, ice cream, etc.). During the second twenty-four hours the patient may have only a clear liquid diet, and is encouraged to drink extra fluids. (Clear liquids, such as soft drinks, clear soups, gelatin desserts, water, etc., are acceptable.) This further decreases any residue in the colon.

Cathartics should not be used for the patient who is recovering from an acute attack of diarrheal illness, or who has more than four bowel movements per day. The patient should be given an enema on the day of the examination after the forty-eight-hour liquid diet. The enema should consist of approximately one quart of warm tap water administered two hours before the endoscopic procedure, so that most of the fluid will be evacuated prior to examination.

Those patients having two to four loose bowel movements per day will still have some residual fecal material in the bowel on the day of the examination and should be given five ounces of citrate of magnesia on the night prior to the examination. Two tap water enemas should be taken on the morning of the examination, in addition to the liquid diet.

Patients who have a normal bowel pattern (usually those undergoing periodic surveillance for precancerous changes in ulcerative colitis) should be given ten ounces of citrate of magnesia on the day before colonoscopy, in addition to the liquid diet and tap water enemas given about two hours before the procedure.

Most colonoscopic examinations are now performed in out-patient clinics or doctors' offices, and patients may return home immediately following the examination. Since medications such as Valium and Demerol will be given intravenously to relax the patient and minimize discomfort, a friend or relative should accompany the patient home. The patient should not drive for at least twelve hours following the intravenous administration of these medications.

The Examination

Colonoscopy reveals many visual features that can help the physician in making a differential diagnosis between ulcerative colitis and Crohn's disease. These include loss of the normal fold pattern in the colon, ulcerations, and any lesion along the wall of the colon. In addition, the physician may also be able to recognize alteration in the vascular pattern caused by blood vessels in the colon, or gradations in color that may be a determinant in diagnosis, as well as obtain biopsy specimens.

As discussed earlier, the major reason for performing a colonoscopic examination in patients with inflammatory bowel disease is to investigate more thoroughly an abnormality seen on a previous barium enema X-ray examination. For example, an X ray cannot distinguish between various types of polyps (elevations above the surface lining of the colon). These include the benign polyps with a potential for growing into cancer, known as adenomas, and nonmalignant pseudopolyps with no cancer potential. Both types are often seen in IBD. Some patients with inflammatory bowel disease may also develop polyps similar to those that occur in people without colon disease. X rays may also reveal cancerous polyps. Most of the time the radiologist will be able to distinguish between cancerous and benign polyps, but may not be able to distinguish whether a benign polyp is an adenoma or a pseudopolyp. When this difficulty arises, colonoscopy may help because it allows the physician to see the polyps and the surrounding area in question, and to take a biopsy.

LOOKING FOR CANCER
IN ULCERATIVE COLITIS

Cancer occurs in patients with ulcerative colitis more frequently than in patients with Crohn's disease. Because of the known cancer potential of ulcerative colitis, attempts have been made to identify the particular patients in this high-risk category who may, at some future date, develop cancer. Malignancy in ulcerative colitis may go through a "precancer" phase, during which characteristic microscopic changes occur in the individual cells lining the colon. These early cellular changes are termed *dysplasia* by the pathologist, and the presence of dysplasia in the colon alerts the physician to the possibility that a subsequent carcinoma might develop. Multiple biopsies of the colon are necessary because of the patchy nature of the dysplasia. Frequently, the endoscopist may not be able to identify an abnormal area of the bowel, but the pathologist will be able to see early cellular changes that may put that patient into a high-risk category. An experienced pathologist is essential for the accurate diagnosis of dysplasia. Second-opinion review of the biopsy by other pathologists is standard practice. Dysplasia in the colon is a reason for repeating colonoscopic examination and biopsies in three months to reconfirm its presence and to grade its severity. A full discussion of the risk of cancer in IBD will be found in Chapter 9.

GASTROSCOPY

Crohn's disease may affect the stomach and duodenum (the uppermost section of the small intestine) as well as other parts of the digestive tract. Under these circumstances, gastroscopy may be indicated. A gastroscope is an instrument similar to the colonoscope that is passed through the mouth to inspect directly the lining of the esophagus, stomach, and duodenum. The instrument is shorter and thinner than the colonoscope but has the same features. The examination is relatively safe and can be accomplished in less than one half-hour. There is little discomfort associated with the gastroscopic examination, but patients are usually given sedative medication to allay apprehension and decrease the gag reflex that may occur in the unsedated patient.

5

SYSTEMIC

MANIFESTATIONS

The main symptoms of IBD—diarrhea, bleeding, and abdominal pain—arise from the intestinal tract. In addition to these local effects, IBD can cause signs or symptoms separate from the bowel. Some of these are quite common and not very specific—for example, weakness, loss of appetite, fever, irritability, or depression. These generalized symptoms are common to nearly all chronic illnesses, and usually respond to treatment of the underlying condition. In addition, several more specific complications are seen in some patients with IBD. For example, certain types of arthritis, skin conditions, inflammations of the eye, and liver dysfunction are recognized as complications of IBD. These conditions are sometimes referred to as "extraintestinal" or "systemic" complications of IBD, since the target organs are separate from the bowel.

In most patients, these bothersome conditions disappear entirely when the disease is brought under control. Rarely, they may precede the bowel disease by several weeks or even months. Although the exact causes of these complications of IBD are not known, it appears that the patient's immune response to the bowel disease triggers inflammation in other parts of the body.

FREQUENCY OF OCCURRENCE
IN IBD PATIENTS

Several large studies indicate that approximately one-third of all IBD patients will develop a problem outside the bowel sometime during the course of their illness. Although Crohn's disease and ulcerative colitis differ in the way they affect the bowel, they are quite similar in the kinds of systemic complications they cause. In fact, the incidence of these complications is about the same for both diseases. In most patients the complications are relatively mild and are more of a nuisance than anything else. Only rarely, probably in less than 1 percent of cases, do complications themselves cause major difficulties. It is important for both patient and doctor to recognize these complications so that prompt treatment can be started.

CAUSES OF
EXTRAINTESTINAL COMPLICATIONS

The cause of complications outside the bowel in IBD patients is not entirely clear. The most likely possibility is some derangement of the patient's immune system, the major defense mechanism of the body, which triggers inflammation in other organs and tissues. As mentioned previously, patients with IBD produce antibodies against bacteria in the colon, and against their own intestinal cells. This means that the defense system of the body, which usually directs antibodies against harmful bacteria and toxins, for some reason attacks the patient's own tissues. The presence of antibodies or other defense mechanisms directed against the self is called autoimmunity. Several other diseases, including lupus erythematosus and rheumatoid arthritis, are called autoimmune diseases because in these disorders damage to various organs may be caused by antibodies or lymphocytes directed against the patient's own tissues.

The scenario in IBD might work something like this. The first step is inflammation of the bowel caused by Crohn's disease or ulcerative colitis. Continued inflammation leads to damaging the cells lining the bowel. The host defenses are now activated to attack any microorganisms attempting to cross the damaged bowel. Antibodies are produced against these invaders, and probably also against damaged intestinal cells. If the bowel inflammation continues, these antibodies may eventually circulate throughout the body, settle in other organs, and lead to complications there.

Obviously, this oversimplified explanation raises more questions than it answers. Why do only some patients with IBD develop complications in other organs? Why does one patient develop arthritis, while another may be troubled with skin lesions? Why does the immune system appear to attack the patient's tissues? These questions cannot be answered now, but there is hope that our research efforts over the next few years will solve these puzzles. Great progress has been made recently in the field of immunology, and it is only a matter of time until these advances will be applied to IBD research.

ARTHRITIS IN IBD

Involvement of the joints is the single most common

complication of IBD, affecting about 25 percent of all patients. The most common joint complaint is arthralgia, or aching of the joints. This symptom is not to be confused with arthritis, or inflammation of the joints, in which the joints become swollen, red, and tender. Arthralgias are not a serious complication and usually disappear as the IBD improves. Aspirin or acetominophen (Tylenol, etc.) may provide relief for arthralgias, but should not be taken unless recommended by your doctor, especially if you are taking other drugs.

Several different types of arthritis associated with IBD have been described. The most common type (mono-arthritis) attacks one joint at a time, usually the knee or ankle. The patient may note swelling, redness, and pain, especially on arising in the morning, and may limp if the arthritis is severe. This one-joint arthritis typically comes and goes with the bowel disease: when the ulcerative colitis or Crohn's disease is active, the arthritis is active. Sometimes it may precede the bowel disease by a week or two, or even by several months or years.

The treatment of this kind of arthritis is aimed primarily at the bowel disease. Your doctor may prescribe sulfasalazine or prednisone to control the diarrhea or bleeding, and as these medicines start to work, the arthritis will lessen, too. Permanent joint deformity ("crippling arthritis") does not occur in this situation; complete recovery is the rule.

Another type of arthritis involves several joints and moves around from joint to joint (polyarthritis). This type can be confused with other types of migrating arthritis conditions such as rheumatoid arthritis or rheumatic fever. Like the single-joint arthritis, polyarthritis generally comes and goes with the bowel disease, and does not lead to permanent joint damage.

Arthritis of the lower spine and pelvis, or sacroileitis, is also quite common in IBD patients. This is usually quite mild, causing low back pain or stiffness from time to time, especially in the morning. A more severe form of spinal arthritis, called ankylosing spondylitis, is a rare complication of IBD. Spondylitis attacks the spine, and to a lesser extent the knees, hips, and shoulders. In more severe cases the spine may become rigid, leading to limitation of movement and considerable disability. This type of arthritis, unlike the others, does not necessarily get better when the bowel improves, and requires intensive medical treatment with nonsteroid anti-inflammatory drugs as well as physiotherapy.

SKIN DISORDERS IN IBD

The skin disturbances seen in IBD patients are also thought to arise from immune factors, although proof for this theory is lacking. One of the more common skin problems is erythema nodosum, which means "red bumps." These red tender nodules, about a half-inch to one inch across, occur most often over the shins or ankles. Erythema nodosum usually crops up when the bowel disease flares, or sometimes just before a flare-up. It is quite common in young women with Crohn's disease or ulcerative colitis and distinctly rare in older patients. Other diseases can cause erythema nodosum, but its occurrence in patients with known IBD should alert the doctor and patient to the likelihood of increased activity of bowel disease. Erythema nodosum is not disfiguring or chronic, and disappears completely when the bowel disease is brought under control.

A more troublesome but fortunately quite rare skin problem in IBD patients is pyoderma, which means "pus in the skin." Pyoderma causes deep, chronic ulcers on the shins or ankles, and occasionally over the calf, and may occur after injury to the area. Again, younger women are more likely to develop this condition than older patients or men. The ulcers heal slowly as the IBD is brought under control, although skin grafting is occasionally required to cover the denuded area.

Stomatitis, or inflammation of the mouth, is another manifestation of IBD. Aphthous stomatitis (canker sores, cold sores) is a shallow ulceration inside the mouth, usually between the gum and lower lip, or along the side or base of the tongue. These painful sores occur more commonly in Crohn's disease than in ulcerative colitis, and usually subside as the bowel disease is brought under control. Local application of corticosteroid-containing ointment may be used to relieve pain, but is not always effective. Local anesthetic agents in a special adhering ointment may also be useful.

EYE PROBLEMS

Inflammation of the eye occasionally occurs in patients with IBD, again usually during or just before a flare-up of the bowel disease. The typical complaint is a red painful eye, and photophobia, or "fear of light" because light aggravates the discomfort. Rarely, vision may be impaired. This complication is often self-limiting and gradually disappears when Crohn's disease or colitis is brought under control. Therapy usually consists of topical (local) medication, but may require oral medication directed at the bowel disease. Inflammation of the eye should always be evaluated by a physician, especially if it lasts for more than twenty-four hours.

LIVER DISEASE IN IBD

The liver is a digestive organ in the abdomen; it communicates with the bowel by way of the bile duct, which carries bile from the liver to the upper small intestine. Neither Crohn's disease nor ulcerative colitis involves the liver directly, but inflammation of the liver or the bile ducts can occur in IBD patients. Liver complications are usually quite minor, and in general do not cause symptoms. The presence of more significant liver problems may be suspected if a patient develops jaundice and/or pain in the right upper abdomen over the liver. Other symptoms that might suggest liver problems are itching, fever, a dragging sensation in the abdomen due to liver enlargement, or abdominal swelling. A few simple blood tests will usually reveal the presence of liver disease, but occasionally liver biopsy or specialized tests such as X rays, ultrasound, or liver scans, are necessary for accurate diagnosis.

The most common liver problem in IBD patients is fatty liver, in which the liver cells become infiltrated and swollen with fat. This does not result from a diet rich in fatty foods, but rather from a disturbance in liver metabolism that may be associated with prednisone therapy and poor nutrition. This condition is usually mild and resolves with treatment of the bowel disease and improved nutrition.

Inflammation of the bile ducts, or cholangitis, is a rare complication of IBD. The inflammation may lead to partial blockage of the ducts, resulting in jaundice, and infection of the bile. Bile duct inflammation may respond to medical treatment aimed at the IBD, but fortunately this complication does not progress rapidly. Rarely, cancer of the bile ducts may develop for unknown reasons in persons with long-standing IBD.

Gallstones are quite common in people of the United States and Western Europe, owing to our diet rich in meat, dairy products, and fried foods. In patients with Crohn's disease of the ileum, gallstones are even more common than in the general population, because the diseased ileum is unable to absorb bile salts, which are in turn required to solubilize cholesterol in bile. When cholesterol precipitates out of the bile, cholesterol gallstones result. In many patients with gallstones, pain or other complications may require removal of the gall bladder. Gallstones are diagnosed by oral cholecystogram X rays or a sonogram of the gall bladder.

MISCELLANEOUS COMPLICATIONS

Although the kidney is not involved directly by inflammatory bowel disease, it may be affected secondarily. Kidney stones occur more commonly in IBD patients whose disease involves the small intestine, and especially in those who have had partial removal of the small intestine. These patients tend to excrete more oxalate in the urine, and this type of mineral salt in excess can cause kidney stones. Dehydration secondary to chronic diarrhea also contributes to kidney stone formation in patients with IBD. If you develop an oxalate stone, your doctor will probably recommend an increase in fluid intake and avoidance of oxalate-rich foods or drinks such as spinach, beets, turnips, tea, and cola.

The urine tube, or ureter, which carries urine from the kidney to the urinary bladder, may become partially blocked in certain patients with Crohn's disease. The usual cause is a mass of inflamed bowel that presses on the ureter and partially obstructs it. An X-ray test called an intravenous pyelogram (IVP) is needed to diagnose this condition.

Some patients with Crohn's disease of the small bowel have reduced absorption of food and nutrients, especially when a considerable portion of the small bowel has been removed surgically. Loss of three feet or more of the small bowel can result in impaired absorption of nutrients, and

51

diarrhea. A low-fat diet and antidiarrheal drugs may be beneficial. Since vitamin B-12 is absorbed in the ileum, some patients with Crohn's disease of the ileum, especially those who have undergone resection of the ileum, may develop vitamin B-12 deficiency. This is easily treated by monthly injections of this essential vitamin. Deficiencies of vitamins A, D, and K may also be supplemented either by tablets or injection.

SUMMARY

Approximately one-third of patients with IBD will have complications in an organ outside the bowel. These complications are usually mild, and disappear when the bowel disease is treated. Only rarely do they overshadow the bowel symptoms or require surgery for their control. Moreover, the occurrence of an extraintestinal manifestation does not necessarily indicate deterioration of the bowel, or a poor prognosis. Ongoing research on the role of immune features in inflammatory bowel disease should provide a better understanding of these complications and more effective treatment of IBD in general.

PART II
Treating the Diseases

6

MEDICATIONS AND
THEIR SIDE EFFECTS

At present, there is no medical (non-surgical) cure for Crohn's disease or ulcerative colitis. The most important goal of treatment is to control the inflammatory reaction in order to diminish diarrhea, abdominal pain, fever, rectal bleeding, and loss of appetite and weight. If medical treatment is successful, these signs and symptoms of disease activity should decrease and the disease may go into remission. Remissions may last a few weeks to many years.

Currently, medical treatment generally consists of the use of one or more anti-inflammatory drugs. The two most important drugs in this group are sulfasalazine and corticosteroids. In addition, some physicians have recommended the use of immunosuppressive drugs and/or antibiotics. Usually medications are administered by mouth, but some drugs are beneficial when given rectally as a suppository, enema, or foam. In severe illnesses, medications may be administered either by intramuscular injection or by intravenous infusion.

SULFASALAZINE

Sulfasalazine (Azulfidine) is probably one of the most widely used medications in the treatment of inflammatory bowel disease. Even after many years of use, the specific way in which the drug acts is not fully understood. Sulfasalazine consists of two parts: a sulfa preparation (sulfapyridine) and an aspirinlike drug called acetylsalicylic acid. In order for the drug to be effective, bacteria in the colon must first break the bond linking its two components. Since other sulfa preparations given alone are not very effective, the sulfa component is probably not responsible for the beneficial effects of sulfasalazine.

Once liberated from the parent compound, sulfapyridine is absorbed systemically and may be responsible for the unpleasant side effects that often occur when sulfasalazine is administered. Research suggests that the active part of sulfasalazine is acetylsalicylic acid, which undergoes further change in the intestinal tract to 5-aminosalicylic acid (5-ASA) and other metabolites (products). It is by acting topically that 5-ASA suppresses inflammatory reactions in colon tissue; very little is absorbed into the bloodstream. Very high concentrations of 5-ASA can be found in the stools of persons taking sulfasalazine. One recent study has demonstrated the effectiveness of locally administered 5-ASA suppositories in reducing rectal inflammation in ulcerative colitis. Unfortunately, 5-ASA given alone orally is broken down before it reaches the inflammation site. Since the major side effects appear to be due to sulfapyridine, investigations are now underway to link 5-ASA with an inert compound so that bacterial action in the colon will liberate the active drug with none of the unpleasant side effects of sulfapyridine.

Sulfasalazine is available in tablet form as 0.5 gram. It is also available as an enteric-coated tablet (which allows it to dissolve slowly, preventing stomach irritation) and as a liquid suspension. The drug is most effective in patients with mild to moderately severe ulcerative colitis. Many physicians administer the drug by starting with one tablet per day, increasing the dose by a tablet until a total daily dosage of 4.0 grams is achieved, i.e. eight tablets daily administered in divided doses, usually after meals. The drug usually takes one to two weeks to work.

Once the symptoms are under control, the dose of sulfasalazine can be reduced. Many physicians then place patients on a "maintenance" dose of the drug for long periods. Some studies have shown that in addition to reducing the acute inflammation of ulcerative colitis, sulfasalazine can also prevent relapses of this disease.

Controlled studies have shown that sulfasalazine is also of value in treating flare-ups of Crohn's colitis and ileocolitis. It is apparently less helpful in treating disease confined to the ileum, according to results published by the National Cooperative Crohn's Disease Study. The drug is probably not helpful in preventing recurrences of Crohn's disease after surgery.

SIDE EFFECTS OF SULFASALAZINE

The most common side effects of treatment with sulfasalazine are nausea and headache, which seem to be related to the dose and to the way in which the body metabolizes the drug. These reactions can be diminished by reducing the dosage by 0.5 gram increments daily. Another side effect is a rash which may be caused by sensitivity to the sulfa component. When this occurs, the drug may be discontinued. Desensitization to sulfa may then be undertaken by starting with one-quarter of a tablet daily, increasing the dose gradually over a long period of time. Side effects of sulfasalazine appear to be lessened when corticosteroid preparations are being used simultaneously. Since anemia and low white blood cell counts may occur during sulfasalazine administration, physicians often arrange for a complete blood count to be performed at regular intervals. Sulfasalazine may interfere with the absorption of other drugs, and it is therefore important to inform your physician about other medications you are taking.

Sulfasalazine has been available for many years and is felt to be a safe drug, even with long-term use. It has even been demonstrated as safe for use during pregnancy: a recent national study found no adverse effects caused by sulfasalazine in pregnant women or their newborn infants. The pharmaceutical industry is now attempting to develop a preparation containing 5-ASA that can be taken orally and delivered in therapeutically effective concentrations to the inflamed colon. This should reduce side effects caused by the sulfa component and, it would be hoped, maintain the anti-inflammatory properties attributed to the 5-ASA portion.

CORTICOSTEROIDS

Corticosteroids are widely used in treating all forms of Crohn's disease and ulcerative colitis. These are very potent agents that can relieve many of the signs and symptoms of active inflammatory bowel disease as well as some of the systemic manifestations such as arthritis and inflammation of the skin and eyes.

We do not fully understand the manner in which this group of drugs exerts its beneficial effects. While the anti-inflammatory properties of corticosteroids are probably the most important in treating IBD, they appear to have immunosuppressive actions as well. In acute disease, corticosteroids often cause dramatic improvement with reduction of fever, amelioration of pain, cessation of diarrhea and bleeding, and an increase in well-being and appetite. Inflammatory masses may shrink, and partial intestinal obstruction caused by edema (swelling) may also be relieved by the use of these medications. Controlled studies such as the National Cooperative Crohn's Disease Study have demonstrated the efficacy of corticosteroids in the short-term treatment of acute Crohn's disease. Unfortunately, these and other studies have not found low-dose "maintenance" corticosteroids useful in preventing flare-ups of either Crohn's disease or ulcerative colitis, or in preventing recurrence of Crohn's disease after surgery.

The most commonly used corticosteroids include prednisone and prednisolone. These drugs are synthetic agents which closely resemble the hormone cortisol, released from the adrenal cortex. A related medication that is sometimes used is corticotropin (ACTH). Corticotropin is a hormone secreted by the pituitary gland which stimulates the release of cortisol from the adrenal gland. This drug may be used as an intramuscular or intravenous preparation.

Corticosteroids given by mouth are absorbed in the small intestine. If an individual is unable to take oral feedings, corticosteroids can be given intravenously or intramuscularly. They may also be given in enema form, as suppositories, or as foam introduced directly into the rectum. If there is active inflammation of the rectum, relatively little of this medication is absorbed, and whatever benefit occurs is the result of topical action. If the rectal mucous membrane is less inflamed, perhaps 30 to 40 percent of the administered dosage is absorbed systemically.

Corticosteroids are usually begun in doses high enough to induce a remission or reduction of active symptoms, and then tapered slowly over weeks and months. The dose and duration of steroid therapy depends upon how sick the patient is and how he or she responds to the drug. While corticosteroids are given most often on a daily basis (and at first several times during the day), with some patients who have responded well to them they are effective when given every other day. This may be a particularly helpful way to administer corticosteroids in the child or adolescent, since giving the drug every other day markedly diminishes side effects such as growth impairment, delay in sexual maturation, and adrenal suppression. This method of administering steroids may be ineffective, however, when IBD is very active.

SIDE EFFECTS OF CORTICOSTEROIDS

Corticosteroid preparations may cause a host of side effects that can be quite distressing to the person experiencing them. In addition to the side effects already discussed, others include rounding of the face (facial "mooning"), acne, increased appetite, weight gain, red marks or blotches on the skin, and increased body and facial hair in both sexes. Less commonly, there may be thinning of the bones, peptic ulcer, diabetes, hypertension, and significant personality changes. Side effects such as these usually diminish as the dose is reduced, and disappear when the medication is discontinued. Patients on prolonged steroid therapy should be evaluated by an eye doctor regularly because of the possibility that cataracts or glaucoma might develop.

While the list of these side effects is long, the majority of patients who take corticosteroids benefit from their use. The physician must weigh the therapeutic benefits of corticosteroids against their potential side effects in deciding upon a course of therapy. In Crohn's disease complicated by intra-abdominal abscess, complex sinus tracts, or fistulas, steroid therapy requires considerable experience and caution. Many physicians faced with complications such as these strive to taper the dosage of steroids to avoid the possibility that infections might develop while steroids are being used.

IMMUNOSUPPRESSIVES

In the late 1950s and early 1960s it was fashionable to believe that most diseases of unknown etiology were "auto-immune"—that is, caused by an attack of the patient's own antibody defense mechanisms against internal organs. Indeed, in 1959, Swedish scientists had reported that antibodies against colon tissues could be found circulating in the blood of certain patients with ulcerative colitis. Doctors therefore reasoned that ulcerative colitis as well as other "autoimmune" diseases should be improved by treatment with antimetabolite drugs—chemical variants of basic building blocks of cell nuclei that would infiltrate normal antibody-producing cells and poison them at critical stages in their metabolism, thus suppressing this destructive immune response.

The first trial of this theory was conducted in Australia over 20 years ago. Dr. R. H. D. Bean treated one of his ulcerative colitis patients with the antimetabolite, 6-mer-captopurine (6-MP). The patient experienced a prompt and dramatic remission which lasted throughout two years of treatment and continued for months thereafter. In 1962, Bean published an enthusiastic account of this experience in the *Medical Journal of Australia.* When he provided an equally favorable follow-up report of seven cases in 1966, the era of immunosuppressive trials for inflammatory bowel disease was launched. Ulcerative colitis, however, is readily curable by surgery. Moreover, both the disease and its antimetabolite treatment are feared to carry some potentially increased risks of cancer (see Chapter 9). For both these reasons, there has not been widespread enthusiasm for immunosuppressive therapy of ulcerative colitis. We will return to this issue later in this chapter. But Crohn's disease has been another story. This chronic, stubborn disease is not so amenable to surgical cure. Doctors and patients alike are willing to grasp harder at medical treatments. Immunosuppressive therapy has therefore become a major issue in Crohn's disease.

The first landmark of immunosuppressive therapy in Crohn's disease was established in London in 1969, under the leadership of Bryan Brooke, an eminent surgeon who invented the modern ileostomy. Six of Brooke's patients were treated for six months with azathioprine (Imuran), a close chemical relative of 6-MP, and all six experienced clinical improvement. Soon after the publication of Brooke's report in the popular British medical journal, *The Lancet,* doctors at many other medical centers jumped onto the immunosuppressive bandwagon. Fifteen published reports appeared quickly. Each was purely anecdotal, described only one or at best a handful of cases, provided only a short follow-up, failed to consider the effects of additional treatment being given at the same time, and included no control experiments. This last defect was the most serious. Since Crohn's disease often follows an unpredictable course of spontaneous exacerbations and remissions, and since patients and doctors both very much want to believe in the effectiveness of whatever treatment they are using, any new drug being tried out may appear beneficial, at least temporarily, as a combined result of power of suggestion, wishful thinking, and coincidence. Yet even amid the potentially misleading data from all these uncontrolled studies, two intriguing patterns could be discerned. First, occasional patients experienced remissions so striking and dramatic that it was not easy to explain them all away as purely due to "placebo effect" or bias. Second, two types of clinical response to azathioprine seemed to occur with consistency throughout the varied reports: closure of fistulas and reduction of steroid requirement.

For these reasons, it was soon recognized that properly controlled scientific studies were needed to explore the real value of immunosuppressives in Crohn's disease. In a controlled "double blind" study designed to avoid bias, patients are randomly assigned to receive either the new treatment, the alternate treatment, or a placebo (inert substance), with neither the patients nor their doctors knowing which treatment is being administered until after the study is over and the clinical results recorded. In the first half of the 1970s, five such double blind trials were conducted, comparing azathioprine to placebo in nearly 100 patients with Crohn's disease. The conclusions were not identical, but certain clues to potential benefits of azathioprine kept emerging. In three of the five studies, azathioprine was statistically significantly better than placebo in inducing remissions of disease, reducing steroid requirements, or promoting subjective improvement in the patients. In the remaining two studies, the overall differences between azathioprine and placebo treatment did not reach statistical significance, but only the patient groups receiving azathioprine experienced any dramatic remissions and avoided any surgery. In yet another study, patients in remission on azathioprine experienced a one-year relapse rate of 41 percent when switched to placebo, versus only 5 percent when maintained on azathioprine.

Then, in 1977, the long-awaited results of the National Cooperative Crohn's Disease Study (NCCDS) were published (*Gastroenterology,* October 1979). The NCCDS gave good grades to sulfasalazine and prednisone. Azathioprine, too, scored better than placebo, but not sufficiently better to achieve levels of conventional statistical significance (in which statistical analysis must demonstrate no greater than

5 percent probability that any difference in results might have occurred simply by chance). This report threatened to close the book forever on the immunosuppressive treatment of Crohn's disease. But in 1972, a larger study had been launched in New York, spearheaded by Drs. D. H. Present and B. I. Korelitz of the Mount Sinai and Lenox Hill hospitals. This study, which was completed in 1979 and published in *The New England Journal of Medicine* in 1980, reached a different conclusion. Seventy-two patients were treated with either 6-MP or placebo for no less than six months, and in most cases for a total of two years. Clinical improvement occurred in 67 percent of patients on 6-MP versus 8 percent on placebo. (Statistical analysis indicates that the probability of this difference having occurred purely by chance is less than one in ten thousand.) Of patients treated with 6-MP, 50 percent were able to discontinue steroids altogether, and another 25 percent could reduce them, versus 15 percent on placebo. Fistulas healed completely in 31 percent of patients on 6-MP, versus 6 percent on placebo.

The benefits of 6-MP, therefore, were unmistakable, but they were not unalloyed. They took a long time to appear, requiring more than three months in a third of the patients and over four months in 20 percent. Moreover, fully 10 percent of patients on 6-MP experienced some adverse side effects of the medication, including fevers, bone marrow suppression, and pancreatitis. To be sure, all side effects proved completely reversible upon discontinuing the drug; there were no permanent injuries, malignancies nor deaths. The fact remains, however, that the immunosuppressive drugs azathioprine and 6-MP are potentially dangerous and require close monitoring of patients' blood counts and clinical condition. They should be avoided during pregnancy, and could conceivably have long-term side effects that are still not fully appreciated. At present, their use is generally recommended only in cases of chronic high-dose steroid dependency, stubborn fistulas unresponsive to conservative measures, and severe debilitating diseases not amenable to corrective surgery or any other simpler treatment. These drugs are no cure-all nor easy solution, but they now have a place in the armamentarium of physicians who wage an uneven battle against Crohn's disease.

Fortunately, the battle against ulcerative colitis is not quite so uneven. Steroids may be more effective here than in Crohn's disease, and in any event colectomy is always available as the ultimate weapon. However, several published studies and considerable clinical experience do point to a limited role for immunosuppressive therapy in ulcerative colitis, too. Every so often, a patient is virtually disabled by severe proctitis or proctosigmoiditis. The disease is uncontrolled by acceptable doses of steroids, yet the patient is not so sick as to require total proctocolectomy and ileostomy. In certain of these cases, in which the patient is desperate but where radical surgical treatment seems even worse than the limited disease, there might be a role for immunosuppressive therapy. As in most such therapeutic dilemmas, decisions should be reached in open partnership between patient and physician, with the risks and benefits carefully weighed for all therapeutic options.

METRONIDAZOLE (FLAGYL)

Metronidazole is a drug that has been used effectively for over twenty years against a wide variety of parasitic and bacterial infections. The history of its more recent use in Crohn's disease parallels that of immunosuppressives: an initial report of one doctor's experience with a few patients, a subsequent spate of reports of uncontrolled series, and finally some double blind trials. In the case of metronidazole, the story began in Sweden in 1975 with a report by Dr. B. O. Ursing describing favorable experience in five patients with Crohn's disease. Soon thereafter, results of metronidazole treatment were reported in more than 200 Crohn's disease patients around the world, with 70 to 80 percent of them allegedly showing benefit. Besides an overall improvement in clinical condition, occasional notice was taken of remarkable healing of fistulous disease around the anus. Interest in metronidazole was particularly stimulated in the United States in 1980 when Dr. Leslie Bernstein and his colleagues described dramatic improvement in perianal Crohn's disease in 100 percent of patients treated with this drug.

Controlled studies to date have not invariably confirmed with statistical significance the overall effectiveness of metronidazole in treating Crohn's disease, but there have been too many individual instances of dramatic responses—especially regarding perianal fistulas—to be ignored. Most recently, a large multicenter nationwide study in Sweden has demonstrated that metronidazole has clinical and anti-inflammatory activity in Crohn's disease at least as great as or greater than that of sulfasalazine.

Unfortunately, as with immunosuppressive drugs, the price is high—in more than monetary terms. Adverse side effects occur in up to 20 percent of patients. Nausea, and numbness of the hands and feet are particularly troublesome effects, cancer risk and genetic damage are feared though still unproven, and other possible consequences of long-term use are almost completely unknown. Nonetheless, interest in the action of this potent drug is certain to continue in the years ahead.

ANTIBIOTICS

At times, potent antibiotics are required as adjunctive

therapy for septic (infected) complications of Crohn's disease or ulcerative colitis. At other times, however, broad-spectrum antibiotics have been utilized to reduce inflammation presumably caused by bacteria in the wall of the small or large intestine. Thus far, there have been no controlled studies verifying the efficacy of antibiotics for this latter purpose. It should be pointed out that antibiotics themselves may cause side effects, including fungal infections of the vagina, mouth, and perineal areas. Also, as mentioned previously, antibiotic-associated diarrhea may occur when a toxin is produced following the overgrowth of certain bacteria (clostridia) in the colon. Diarrhea that increases after the use of antibiotics should immediately prompt the search for this organism. Fortunately, bacteriology laboratories in most cities now have the technical capacity to identify the presence of the clostridial toxin. If this is found, appropriate therapies are available.

ANTIDIARRHEAL AGENTS

Agents that reduce diarrhea may be very useful in the symptomatic treatment of Crohn's disease. These include diphenoxylate (Lomotil), loperamide (Imodium), paregoric, and codeine. These drugs alter the activity of smooth muscle in the wall of the gut. Antidiarrheal agents can also be of benefit to patients who have had a resection of the terminal ileum and part of the colon, or to patients with an ileostomy, but have little effect in curbing diarrhea caused by active rectal disease. As a consequence, there is urgency and the passage of small amounts of stool at frequent intervals. If an antidiarrheal agent is used in the mistaken notion that this type of diarrhea can be controlled, a fecal impaction may be created above the narrowed, inflamed rectal segment.

Caution is advisable when prescribing antidiarrheal

agents in patients with very active inflammatory bowel disease. They may cause toxic dilatation of the colon, which can occur in Crohn's disease as well as in ulcerative colitis. There is also the risk of addiction or dependence.

ANTICHOLINERGIC MEDICATIONS

In addition to codeine, Lomotil, Imodium, and other drugs in this category, anticholinergic medications such as atropine, propantheline (Pro-Banthine), and others are sometimes used in an attempt to reduce cramps or diarrhea in IBD. Anticholinergics temporarily block the transmission of nerve impulses in the bowel, thereby reducing intestinal movement. But their effectiveness is limited, and these drugs, like opiates, may also contribute to the development of toxic dilatation, or may precipitate intestinal obstruction. They also may cause urinary hesitancy and retention, severe dryness of the mouth, visual disturbances, swallowing difficulties, and, on rare occasions, behavioral changes.

CHOLESTYRAMINE

Another drug that may be of help in Crohn's disease is cholestyramine (Questran), a substance that binds bile salts. Cholestyramine is used to control diarrhea associated with extensive disease of the terminal ileum or with surgical resection of less than 100 centimeters of terminal ileum. If severe diarrhea occurs in either clinical situation, the patient may not be absorbing bile salts which, normally absorbed in the terminal ileum, now spill into the colon, causing it to secrete fluid and electrolytes. The result is a watery diarrhea. With cholestyramine binding the bile salts, this form of diarrhea can be prevented. Unfortunately, cholestyramine is somewhat unpalatable and rather expensive. And, if its use is followed by an increase in diarrhea and weight loss, as occasionally happens, it should be discontinued. But when its use results in a marked improvement, it is reasonable to continue cholestyramine treatment under the supervision of a physician. Nonetheless, in selected patients with this specific type of watery diarrhea, its use can result in marked clinical improvement.

SOME DRUGS WITHOUT PROVEN BENEFIT

Coherin

Coherin is a substance extracted from animal pituitary glands near the base of the brain. Some years ago, a physician at a major university medical center began injecting samples of this preparation into his patients with Crohn's disease and ulcerative colitis. Some of his patients felt better after receiving their shots, and this investigator became convinced that he had found a new form of treatment for IBD. Although he was never able to muster scientific evidence for the effectiveness of coherin, he publicized his findings among patients and their physicians. Subsequent investigators at the physician's medical center then conducted a double blind, controlled study of coherin among patients with inflammatory bowel disease, seeking independent verification of the drug's effectiveness. There was none demonstrated. This episode confirms the need for impartial, scientific validation of any therapeutic agents through controlled trials.

Cromolyn

A form of immunosuppression different from antimetabolite therapy is exerted by a drug called cromolyn.

This agent is widely used for inhalation therapy in bronchial asthma. It prevents certain inflammatory cells (known as mast cells) in the bronchial wall from releasing histamine and other chemicals that contribute to the inflammatory process. Efforts have been made to treat ulcerative colitis with this same drug, administered either by mouth or through the rectum. Despite a few early reports of beneficial effect, most results with this treatment have been disappointing.

Other methods of immunosuppressive treatment have included cytoxic drugs, antilymphocyte serum, and plasmapheresis (removal and exchange of the patient's plasma volume in an effort to remove abnormal immune proteins or other deleterious substances). None of these approaches has been shown to be safe and effective.

BCG Vaccine

Many studies of ulcerative colitis and Crohn's disease have raised the suggestion that patients frequently demonstrate deficiencies in certain of their immune functions. For this reason, attempts at therapy in the past decade have included efforts to stimulate, rather than suppress, the immune system. Agents tried have included BCG (an antituberculosis vaccine), transfer factor (an immunostimulating substance extracted from white blood cells), and levamisole (an antiparasite drug with immunostimulating activity). None has proven successful.

7

NUTRITIONAL COMPLICATIONS OF CROHN'S DISEASE AND ULCERATIVE COLITIS

Physicians have known for some time that poor nutrition can complicate the course of inflammatory bowel disease. Until recently, basic mechanisms have been poorly understood and treatment unavailable for inadequately nourished individuals. Thanks to intensive research over the last fifteen to twenty years, much of it sponsored by the National Foundation for Ileitis & Colitis, we can now overcome these barriers and cope with even the most complex and devastating nutritional problems caused by IBD.

In order to understand how inflammatory bowel disease and nutrition interact, we must first review a few basic definitions and physiologic principles. Nutrients, namely fats, carbohydrates, proteins, water, vitamins, minerals, and trace elements are substances we consume to build the body and to fuel and regulate its functions. Nutritional requirements for each person depend on age, sex, size, activity, body temperature, and state of general health. Together these factors determine how rapidly nutrients are used and excreted by the body.

Food enters the body through the mouth, passes through the esophagus to the stomach, and then to the small intestine. In order to be utilized by the body, nutrients must be absorbed from the interior of the small intestine through its lining cells and carried into the bloodstream for distribution to the rest of the body. The composition of foods as they appear at the dinner table is much too complex for the gut to absorb. These foods must undergo digestion, the process by which they are broken down into readily absorbable form. (See Figure 2.) The digestion of fats occurs primarily in the upper half of the small intestine. There, in a sequence that requires the presence of bile salts formed in the liver, chemical compounds called enzymes secreted by the pancreas degrade the fat into smaller particles that the intestinal lining can absorb. Other enzymes from the pancreas are necessary to begin breaking down proteins and carbohydrates into their absorbable building blocks. The process is completed by enzymes that reside in the lining of the small intestine. The absorption of vitamins, minerals, and trace elements is complex and in most cases only partially understood. We know, for example, that fat-soluble vitamin A is assimilated in a manner similar to fat itself. Water-soluble vitamin B-12 must bind with a factor produced in the stomach and travel all the way to the end of the small bowel (terminal ileum) to be taken up at special sites. On the other hand, we know very little about how vitamin K, calcium, magnesium, and zinc are absorbed by the body (Figure 4).

HOW IBD CAN IMPAIR NUTRITION

Inflammatory bowel disease can exert a profound influence on a person's nutritional status. The inflammation *itself* increases the requirements for food. Nutrients, especially

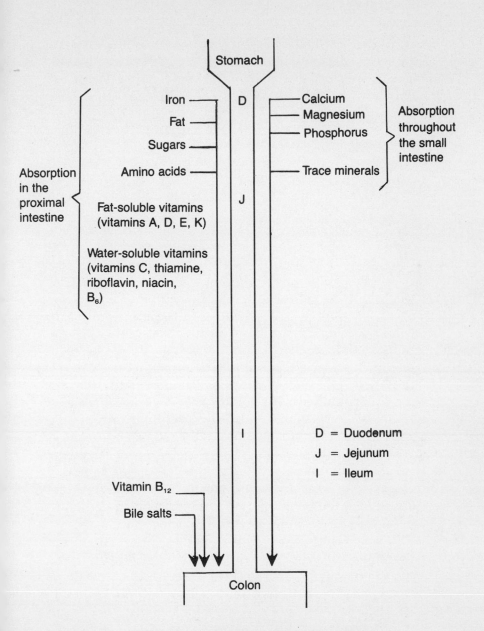

Figure 4. Intestinal absorption of nutrients.

proteans, ooze from the lining of the inflamed bowel and are lost in the stool. By accelerating all metabolic processes, fever raises the need for all nutrients. To make matters worse, a person who feels ill, has fever, pain, or depression, generally has a poor appetite and will not eat enough to meet these increased dietary needs.

Because digestion and absorption take place almost entirely in the small intestine, most nutritional complications in IBD are seen in Crohn's disease, and much less often in ulcerative colitis. Inflammation of the small bowel disrupts the normal absorptive apparatus in the intestinal lining. The location of disease and extent of involvement determine whether or not a particular deficiency will occur. (Table 1 outlines the important symptoms associated with deficiencies found most often in IBD.) If the terminal ileum is diseased, vitamin B-12 absorption will be impaired. More extensive involvement in the small bowel will reduce the milk-sugar digesting enzyme lactase to the point where lactose (milk sugar) will begin to ferment in the small bowel, causing cramps and diarrhea. Inflammation also reduces the functioning surface area of the small intestine; as a result, fats may be poorly absorbed, resulting in cramping and increased amounts of foul-smelling stools (steatorrhea). When severe Crohn's disease involves large areas of the small intestine, or where less than four feet of small intestine are left after operation, the patient may have difficulty absorbing enough nutrients to sustain life, and may require intravenous nutritional support (Table 1).

When Crohn's disease is present in the ileum alone, the nutritional consequences are quite specific. The ileum is the site where the body reabsorbs and recycles bile salts necessary for the absorbtion of fats. Bile salts are normally returned to the liver where they are recycled as bile and reused to digest fats. As mentioned earlier, when bile salts cannot be reabsorbed because of disease in the ileum, they

Table 1. SYMPTOMS ASSOCIATED WITH NUTRITIONAL DEFICIENCIES IN IBD

Symptoms	*Nutritional Deficit*
Generalized malnutrition, as shown by muscle wasting, and growth retardation	Malabsorption of proteins, fats, carbohydrates; insufficient calories
Diarrhea, bloating, gas	Impaired absorption of salt and water caused by carbohydrate and fat malabsorption
Weakness	Anemia; electrolyte (sodium, potassium, bicarbonate, chloride, calcium, magnesium) imbalance
Anemia	Impaired absorption of iron, vitamin B-12 folic acid
Sore mouth and lips	Deficiency of iron and B vitamins
Numbness and tingling	Deficiency of vitamin B-12 or other B vitamins; electrolyte imbalance
Swelling	Protein depletion
Absent menstrual periods	Protein and calorie depletion; rapid loss of weight
Bone pain	Protein depletion; vitamin D and calcium deficiency
Muscle spasms	Electrolyte imbalance (especially, low calcium)
Easy bleeding or bruising	Vitamin K deficiency

pass into the colon where they cause an increase in watery diarrhea. Depletion of bile salts also leads to poor digestion of fats. In addition, influenced by the presence of bile salts and fat malabsorption, the usually impermeable lining of the colon will absorb oxalate, a natural component of many foods. Ordinary concentrations of oxalate are excreted without difficulty by the kidneys, but excess oxalate will crystallize to form kidney stones (calcium oxalate). Patients with a high level of oxalate absorption are advised to avoid foods that are high in oxalate content, such as spinach, cocoa and chocolate, tea, peanuts, and beets.

THE PROBLEM OF BACTERIAL OVERGROWTH

The presence of excess bacteria within the small bowel can cause nutritional problems in Crohn's disease. These organisms normally inhabit the colon in large quantities. In fact, about one-half of the composition of stool is actually bacteria. Spread of bacteria upward to the small intestine is largely prevented by a valve between ileum and colon (the ileocecal valve) and by the downward movement of intestinal contents toward the colon. Partial intestinal obstruction, surgical removal of the ileocecal valve, or the existence of a fistula between the colon and small bowel can allow large quantities of bacteria to populate the small intestine. These bacteria attach themselves to bile salts, making them available for fat digestion. They also bind to vitamin B-12 and prevent its absorption. Bacteria can even produce toxic chemicals which inhibit nutrient absorption by direct damage to the intestinal lining.

NUTRITIONAL PROBLEMS
CAUSED BY TREATMENT

As with any medicine or operation, the treatment of Crohn's

disease and ulcerative colitis may cause unwanted side effects, many with nutritional overtones. For example, when patients with IBD are advised to avoid dairy products, this reduces their calcium and vitamin D intake. Diets low in raw fruits and vegetables (foods which may increase symptoms or obstruct diseased intestine) often lack water-soluble vitamins like folic acid and vitamin C. Malabsorption can result from bowel resection in direct proportion to the length of bowel removed. Prednisone interferes with vitamin D metabolism, impairs calcium absorption, depletes the body's potassium, and increases requirements for proteins and calories. Sulfasalazine inhibits folic acid absorption. Cholestyramine interferes with the absorption of fat and fat-soluble vitamins. This list is not meant to create the impression that the treatment of inflammatory bowel disease is as dangerous as the illness itself! Your physician is well aware of these potential adverse effects of treatment and can prevent or treat them.

TREATING THE NUTRITIONAL PROBLEM

Your doctor commands a substantial array of treatments for the nutritional problems caused by inflammatory bowel disease. Supplementing the diet with proper doses of individual vitamins, minerals, and trace elements will prevent or overcome most deficiencies. Reducing the amount of fat in the diet usually improves the symptoms of malabsorption. Calories lost in this way can be replaced by carbohydrates or medium chain triglycerides, a special kind of fat efficiently absorbed high in the small bowel even without bile and pancreatic enzymes. In the past, lactase deficiency (intolerance to the milk-sugar lactose) has been treated by avoiding milk products. Now there is a commercially available lactase that can be added to bottled milk to predigest lactose into simple absorbable sugars. Bile salt diarrhea can be reduced with resin powders that bind the offending agents so they cannot act on the colon. Cholestyramine (Questran) is the one most commonly employed. Bacterial overgrowth can be checked either by broad-spectrum antibiotics or, when feasible, by surgical correction of the obstruction or fistula responsible for the condition.

Two important new developments, elemental diets and total parenteral nutrition, have dramatically enhanced our ability to treat difficult nutritional problems caused by IBD. Elemental diets are commercially available liquid preparations that contain balanced mixtures of all required nutrients in their most easily absorbable form. Because they need little or no digestion, these preparations are completely assimilated high in the intestine with virtually no residue. Even a person whose small intestine has been drastically shortened by surgery or damaged by inflammation can absorb enough to maintain adequate nutrition. These preparations can be very helpful when intestinal residue is considered harmful, such as in partial obstruction, fistulas, and severe exacerbations of inflammatory activity.

Sometimes it may be impossible or inadvisable for a patient to take *any* nourishment by mouth. For a patient with an especially severe flare-up of Crohn's disease, the physician may wish to prescribe complete bowel rest for several weeks, since diverting food away from the intestine lessens the intensity of the inflammation. Over the several weeks required to achieve bowel rest, however, the patient who is not eating is still expending energy from fever, inflammation, and exudation of body fluids and could become severely malnourished. Similarly, after extensive bowel resection, the patient may have too little intestine remaining to support life, regardless of how much he or she eats. And for the extremely ill patient needing surgery, malnutrition poses the threat of severe complications such as infection. Some form of preoperative nutritional support must be given.

For these types of patients, total parenteral nutrition (TPN, hyperalimentation) has proved lifesaving. This complex and costly technique involves the infusion of concentrated solutions of nutrients in sufficient quantities to maintain or improve the patient's nutritional state. It is a common misconception that patients receiving routine dextrose (sugar) containing intravenous fluids are being "fed" by vein. In fact, these solutions generally contain only a small quantity of sugar and mineral salts and are nutritionally inadequate over long periods of time. If one attempted to put all the essential protein, glucose, salt, minerals, vitamins, and trace elements in the typical intravenous bottle and administer them by the usual arm vein route, the highly concentrated infusion would be intolerably painful and irritating to the vein. For this reason, total parenteral nutrition solutions are usually administered through a catheter inserted into a large central vein, usually the subclavian, just under the collarbone. This catheter can be inserted, with minimal discomfort, by a specialist trained in hyperalimentation. A course of total parenteral nutrition generally lasts for at least a few weeks. Occasionally, longer periods of infusion are necessary—for months, years, or in rare cases, for the remainder of the patient's life. In the past, the complexity and complications of this procedure kept TPN patients in the hospital until the completion of their course. Happily, technology has advanced to the point that even permanent TPN, infused through a surgically implanted catheter, can be managed safely at home. The typical home parenteral nutrition (HPN) patient administers solutions at night during sleep, and during waking hours leads a relatively normal, active life in dependent of the infusion apparatus.

Certain special conditions respond well to treatment by elemental or parenteral feedings. It has been demonstrated that on occasion the prolonged absence of intestinal contents permits the spontaneous closure of Crohn's disease fistulas between bowel and skin. A patient with this complication could become dangerously depleted while waiting for a response to usual medical treatment. TPN or elemental feedings provide the necessary nutrients while the bowel is permitted to rest and the fistulas to heal. In pediatric patients suffering from severe inflammatory bowel disease, growth retardation has been a significant problem, both physically and emotionally. Although impaired growth was once thought to arise mainly from the inflammatory process itself and from the administration of corticosteroids, investigators have demonstrated that inadequate nutrition is the major cause of this distressing complication. Long-term supplementation with either elemental or parenteral feedings have successfully restored many of these children to their normal developmental patterns.

IS THERE A DIET FOR IBD?

The subject of diet therapy for inflammatory bowel disease has aroused enormous interest and controversy; but, in fact, there is little concrete knowledge of exactly how diet affects the course of the disease. For certain specific conditions described previously, there are a variety of specific dietary treatments. For example, where certain deficiencies exist, foods or artificial supplements with high concentrations of the deficient element can be prescribed. Milk products can be eliminated or lactase-digested milk used for lactase deficiency. Low-fat diets are appropriate if there is fat malabsorption. In patients with ileostomies or strictures, foods with large indigestible fibers such as cabbage, corn, nuts, or bran are to be avoided so that obstruction of the stoma or narrowed bowel will not occur. During a flare-up, most physicians will reduce residue or try to rest the bowel with elemental feedings or total parenteral nutrition, depending on the severity of symptoms.

On the other hand, for the patient with mild disease and few or no symptoms, and especially for the patient with disease in remission, there is an active debate among physicians and dieticians about what constitutes an appropriate diet. Should you avoid raw foods and vegetables, spices, roughage, carbonated beverages, or dairy products? Is dietary fiber beneficial or harmful to the person with inflammatory bowel disease? On the basis of clinical experience and training, each gastroenterologist has formulated particular regimens which he or she feels are most beneficial to IBD patients. Only through close communication and cooperation between you and your doctor (and sometimes even through trial and error) can you together find the most beneficial diet for you.

8

THE ROLE OF SURGERY

No one looks forward to any operation. But in seriously ill individuals with Crohn's disease or ulcerative colitis when medical therapy has not relieved symptoms, or when serious complications arise, surgery may provide great relief which cannot be gained in any other way. This chapter will review the reasons for considering surgery in these diseases, the types of surgery available, and some of the complications that occasionally result.

SURGERY FOR
CROHN'S DISEASE

When and why is it necessary to operate in Crohn's disease? In Crohn's disease of the ileum, the two most important reasons to operate are (1) recurrent small bowel obstruction and (2) abscess formation caused by leakage of intestinal contents through sinus tracts that pierce the bowel wall. In Crohn's disease of the colon, surgery may be needed to relieve perforation of the colon, toxic megacolon (an acute dilation of the colon), severe perianal disease, massive bleeding, or unrelieved diarrhea and weight loss. In these cases, surgery can accomplish the following: it can relieve symptoms (such as intestinal obstruction); it removes life-threatening complications (such as an abscess, perforation, or toxic megacolon); it improves the quality of the patient's life by, for instance, alleviating incapacitating perianal disease and persistent diarrhea with weight loss. The most important thing to remember is that surgery is *not* considered a cure for Crohn's disease because the disease does tend to recur after operation.

It is estimated that approximately two-thirds of all patients with Crohn's disease will eventually require surgery and that approximately 40 percent of these may require a second operation. (For this reason, the surgeon will try to conserve as much bowel as possible should another operation be necessary.) Since these figures are based on statistics from teaching hospitals where complicated cases may cluster, it is likely that the inclusion of patients who are not hospitalized would reduce these high figures.

Getting Ready for Surgery

The surgeon is usually consulted early during the management of a patient hospitalized with serious Crohn's disease. In this way, the surgeon can help evaluate individual problems, aid in management during an acute phase of illness, and observe whether a patient is responding to medical therapy. Once the decision to operate is made, the surgeon must prepare the patient so that the operation can be carried out under the best of circumstances. This period of preparation may take from two days in the relatively uncomplicated case to several weeks if the patient is severely malnourished. It is always preferable for a patient to obtain calories and nutrients by mouth if at all possible. For those who cannot absorb the food they eat because of intestinal inflammation, elemental or parenteral feedings may be necessary.

After good nutritional balance has been restored, the operation is far safer for the patient, and the surgeon is frequently in a better position to perform a definitive procedure. During the period of preparation, the acutely ill patient may be taking both antibiotics and corticosteroids. If the patient was receiving steroids before surgery, this medication must be continued both during surgery and during the postoperative period. The reason for this is that the activity of the adrenal gland which makes its own corticosteroids may be suppressed during prior administration of steroids and cannot be relied upon to make sufficient amounts of the hormone during a stressful situation such as surgery. Once beyond the postoperative period, the dosage of steroids can usually be tapered and eventually discontinued.

The final two days of preparation for surgery include bowel cleansing, usually with enemas and irrigations of the colon. As noted previously, strong cathartics are usually not administered by mouth to patients with inflammatory bowel disease because of the possibility of inducing a flare-up. In the twenty-four hours before surgery, patients who do not have an obstruction are usually given oral antibiotics in an attempt to sterilize the contents of the intestine.

There are three major procedures available to the surgeon for the management of Crohn's disease: resection of the bowel, bypass of a diseased segment, and various types of ileostomy. In a patient with reasonable nutritional balance and health, resection if technically feasible is the preferred method of surgery.

Bowel Resection in Crohn's Disease

Resection means removing the diseased bowel and then re-establishing intestinal continuity by suturing the healthy ends together (*anastomosis*). Experience has shown that it is not necessary to remove large areas of normal intestine adjacent to areas of Crohn's disease. As a consequence, only an inch or two of normal-appearing intestine is removed on either side of the diseased intestine during surgery. For example, when the terminal ileum is diseased and requires surgery, the segment is identified and removed, and the healthy ileum is then sewn to the ascending colon. This operation (called a resection with anastomosis) removes the diseased ileum, the lowermost portion of the ascending colon (cecum), and the appendix, which is attached to the cecum. (See Figure 5.) The strategy in this operation is always to retain the maximum amount of normal healthy bowel.

Crohn's disease is characterized by its patchy, segmental nature. Areas of disease are separated by various lengths of normal-appearing bowel. If two areas of bowel are involved with Crohn's disease and are separated by a relatively long segment of normal intestine, the surgeon will not hesitate to remove the two diseased areas, perform two anastomoses, and retain as much normal intestine as possible. When there are several areas of involvement, the surgeon must decide which areas are causing symptoms. Recognizing that it makes no sense to remove every inch of bowel that appears to be involved with Crohn's disease (needlessly sacrificing large amounts of still functioning intestine in the process), most surgeons will leave in place a mildly involved segment of bowel that does not appear to be causing trouble for the patient.

The majority of people with Crohn's disease have involvement of both the small intestine and the colon (ileocolitis).

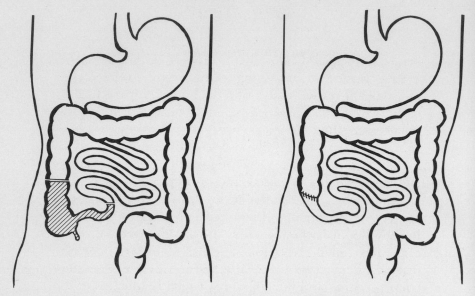

Figure 5. Resection with anastomosis in Crohn's disease. The shaded portion in the diagram on the left represents a diseased segment of ileum and colon. On the right, the diseased bowel has been removed and the surgeon has sutured the remaining ileum and colon together.

Somewhat fewer patients have involvement of the ileum alone, and approximately 15 percent have involvement of the colon alone. Most commonly, the ileocolitis involves the distal (lower) ileum and the ascending (right) colon. There may be disease in various other parts of the colon, but the rectum is often spared. In this case, the surgical procedure is exactly the same as when only the small intestine is involved. The diseased part of ileum and colon are removed and an anastomosis is performed. When skip areas are present, the surgeon must decide whether one or more resections should be carried out. When the rectum is normal, it is almost always possible to restore intestinal continuity by joining the remaining bowel to the rectum, thus avoiding an ileostomy.

When the colon alone is involved, the choice of operation

depends on whether the rectum is normal or diseased. If the rectum is normal, the diseased portion of the colon can be removed, and the ileum can be sewn directly to the remaining colon.

Bypass Operations

Although not performed as often as formerly, bypassing the diseased segment of bowel is an effective operation for Crohn's disease of the lower ileum. In this operation (ileocolostomy with exclusion), the surgeon leaves the diseased bowel segment in place and makes new connection between the healthy ileum and healthy colon. (See Figure 6.) In this way, intestinal contents flow directly from the ileum into the colon, and do not enter the diseased segment, which is sewn shut. Because feces are not passing through it, the diseased segment usually heals, scarring and fibrosis develop, and the segment atrophies, or withers. Once a piece of bowel has been bypassed, it cannot be reconnected even if it heals. It must either be left in place (in the case of patients too ill for further surgery) or subsequently removed. Bypass operations may be performed when the patient is too sick to undergo resection, or when the inflammation is so extensive that an attempt to remove it might jeopardize surrounding structures. Once a very popular form of surgical treatment in Crohn's disease, the bypass operation is performed far less often today because of reports of cancer developing in bypassed loops of bowel many years after surgery.

The Ileostomy in Crohn's Disease

While the two procedures described above are clearly preferable in Crohn's disease, there are situations in which other more extensive procedures are required. For example, when the entire colon and rectum are severely diseased and must be removed, a permanent ileostomy is created.

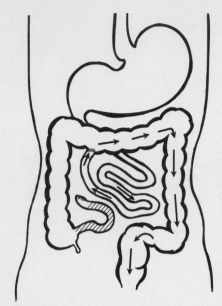

Figure 6. Bypass operation in Crohn's disease. In this diagram, only the terminal ileum is diseased. The surgeon severs the ileum proximal to the diseased area and sutures the remaining ileum to the transverse colon. Intestinal contents then pass directly from the ileum to the transverse colon, bypassing the right colon and the diseased terminal ileum altogether.

This means that after the colon and rectum are removed, the ileum is sewn directly to a new opening on the abdominal wall (stoma), and the bowel waste must empty through it into a bag (Figure 7). A temporary ileostomy can be performed in an emergency situation when the patient is gravely ill with peritonitis from a ruptured abscess or when, in the surgeon's opinion, the patient is so sick that no resection or anastomosis should be attempted. In addition, temporary ileostomy may be performed in conjunction with a colonic resection to protect the suture line during the healing phase. At a later time, once the sutures have healed, the surgeon will close the ileostomy and reconnect the bowel. A two-stage procedure such as this may be necessary in a patient who is depleted or severely ill with serious infection. Today, however, the use of parenteral nutrition allows the surgeon to improve the patient's general condition both before and after surgery, so that this approach may no longer be necessary.

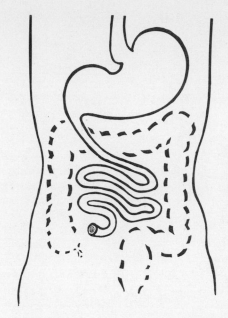

Figure 7. Ileostomy. After surgical removal of colon and rectum, the free end of the ileum is attached to an artificial opening (stoma) created on the lower abdomen. Liquid bowel waste then empties into an appliance fitted over the stoma with a special adhesive.

If Crohn's disease recurs after surgery (as it often does), the surgeon uses the same criteria described above to decide which operation to perform. Resection with reanastomosis is usually the preferred procedure, but depending on the type of recurrence, bypass procedures or ileostomy may also be used.

Surgery for the Complications of Crohn's Disease

The surgical management of fistulas depends upon their location. You will recall that a fistula is an abnormal channel that forms between diseased bowel and another organ or the skin surface. When there is a fistula between the ileum and the colon, the surgeon must determine whether the colon is normal at the site of the fistula or whether it is involved with Crohn's disease. This can usually be determined by barium enema, sigmoidoscopy, or colonoscopy. If the colon is normal, it is usually possible to disconnect the fistulous area, resect the diseased ileum, join the ileum and ascending colon, and repair the colon. If the colon, too, is diseased, it is necessary to remove the involved segment of the colon in addition to resecting the diseased ileum and performing the required anastomoses. When a fistula connects the ileum to the urinary bladder, it is usually possible to separate the bowel from the bladder, close the hole in the bladder, and then remove the diseased ileum. Following closure of a bladder fistula, it is necessary to leave a catheter in the bladder for a period of seven to ten days to ensure healing of that organ.

At times, surgery is performed to treat a large abscess in the abdomen. These abscesses form when a sinus tract pierces the bowel wall permitting intestinal contents and bacteria to enter the otherwise sterile abdominal cavity. Under these circumstances, the surgeon must drain the abscess to reduce the infection. Several weeks later, he or she can remove the diseased bowel with its sinus tract. Otherwise a fistula may develop from the bowel to the skin through the channel occupied by the surgical drain. Such a fistula can be very unpleasant because it discharges liquid fecal waste onto the skin surface.

The Possibility of Complications After Surgery

The major complications following surgery for Crohn's disease are most often caused by infection. Since the bowel wall and the mesentery (supporting structure of bowel) may contain bacteria, wound infections and abscesses may develop after surgery. As a consequence, many surgeons place drains (soft rubber tubes) in the abdomen during surgery which are than removed gradually over a few days with little discomfort. Postoperative management includes the use of a nasogastric (passing through the nose or mouth) tube for drainage of fluid and air from the stomach, intravenous fluids until intestinal function returns, antibiotics, and steroids if the patient has been taking this medication before surgery.

Many patients with Crohn's disease have perianal complications, including abscesses, fissures (cracks), and fistulas. The management of most of these complications is usually conservative and should be handled by medical treatment. However, abscesses must be opened and drained, and painful fistulas often respond well to surgery. In some centers, fistulas and abscesses are drained and dissected to their point of origin (modified Parks operation). This often heals them completely, and does not provoke the underlying Crohn's disease. There are several favorable reports of the use of metronidazole (Flagyl) and immunosuppressive drugs for the management of perianal complications in Crohn's disease, but their long-term role has not yet been clearly defined.

SURGERY FOR ULCERATIVE COLITIS

Ulcerative colitis is a disease that frequently involves the entire colon including the rectum (universal ulcerative colitis). However, the disease may involve only the left side of the colon, and occasionally only the rectum and sigmoid colon (proctosigmoiditis). This group of patients almost never requires surgery.

Because most patients with ulcerative colitis who require surgery have the universal form of the disease, the operation of choice is removal of the entire colon and rectum (total proctocolectomy), and the construction of a standard ileostomy), to collect the fluid fecal waste. With this procedure, patients have to wear a bag constantly since the ileostomy functions almost around the clock. Fortunately, proctocolectomy with ileostomy provides a permanent cure for ulcerative colitis. It does not recur, as may Crohn's disease, after removal of the colon and rectum, and individuals can resume a normal life free of disease.

This operation has stood the test of time. Many patients have had a standard ileostomy for thirty years or more, and have never experienced a day's difficulty. Women have borne children, and conventional ileostomy is no bar to a normal life in all aspects. In fact, many people who have had this operation are leading physically vigorous lives (Figure 8). On the other hand, some patients have great trouble accepting the standard ileostomy and the wearing of a bag, and may delay needed surgery because of this aversion. In the past ten years, several new procedures have been developed which offer new surgical options for these patients.

The Continent (Kock) Ileostomy

The first of these procedures was the development of a continent ileostomy by Dr. Nils Kock of Sweden. In this operation, a total colectomy is performed and the ileum is fashioned in the form of a pouch just behind the ileostomy opening (stoma). The stoma is then positioned exactly level with the skin. A nipple is created (using the patient's own intestine) so that the pouch does not leak gas or stool. The pouch gradually enlarges beneath the skin following surgery, and serves as a reservoir to hold the liquid stool. The patient quickly learns to empty the pouch periodically by inserting a plastic tube into the pouch and draining the liquid stool into the toilet bowl. When the pouch has matured, drainage is required about three to four times per day. If the operation is successful, and over 95 percent of them are, no bag is worn at all. The major complication of this procedure is slippage of the nipple valve so that the patient becomes incontinent. This can be revised surgically to restore continence. While this surgical revision is most often a minor procedure, some patients have required mul-

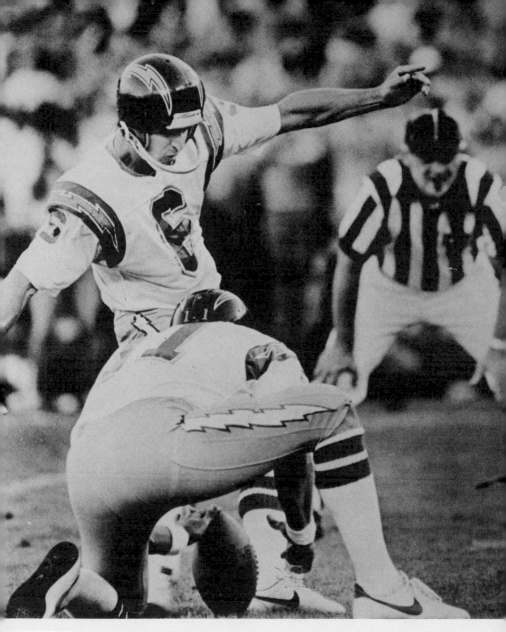

Figure 8. Having an ileostomy does not mean you cannot lead an active life. After the removal of his colon for severe ulcerative colitis, Rolf Benirschke returned to full activity as star placekicker for the San Diego Chargers.

tiple revisions. Most surgeons performing the continent ileostomy prefer to limit its use to ulcerative colitis patients. The reason for this is that if the patient with Crohn's disease develops recurrent ileitis within or near the ileal pouch (a strong likelihood), a considerable amount of ileum may then have to be removed (Figure 9).

Ileoanal Anastomosis

The second major advance in recent years has been the recognition that with patients in whom the rectum is not severely diseased, it is possible to remove its inner lining (mucosal layer), which is the site of the disease, and still preserve the normal muscular tube. In this procedure, a total colectomy is performed and then the mucosal layer is stripped from the rectum, leaving intact and exposing the muscle layers. The ileum is then brought down and sutured to the rectum, just above the anus. (See Figure 10.) This allows the patient to evacuate normally through the anal

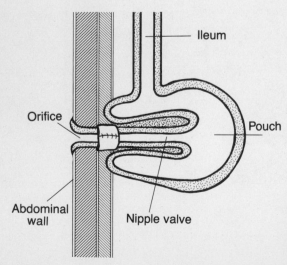

Figure 9. Continent ileostomy. In this operation, the distal ileum is fashioned into a pouch that is then sutured to the interior abdominal wall. The patient learns to remove liquid fecal waste by inserting a thin catheter tube through the orifice and nipple valve into the pouch.

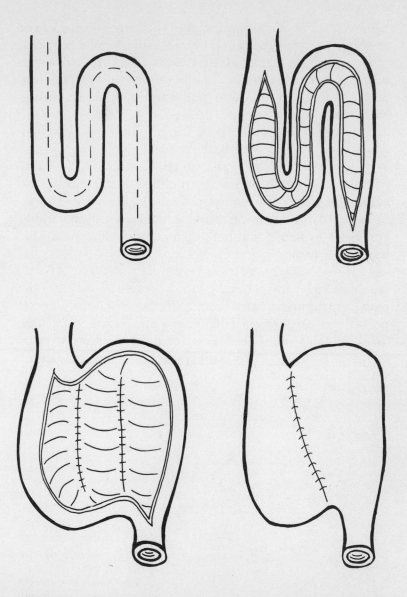

Figure 10. The construction of one type of internal pouch for the ileoanal anastomosis.

sphincters. The procedure includes the creation of a pouch of small intestine above the anastomosis, which acts as a reservoir to hold the liquid stool and reduces the number of bowel movements. When this operation is performed, an ileostomy is performed as a temporary procedure to insure healing of the anastomosis. If all goes well, the temporary ileostomy is closed a few months after initial surgery. When this procedure is successful, the patient may have only four to five stools per day and can be totally continent. Although many ulcerative colitis patients are choosing this type of surgery, no long-term follow-up studies have been done. It will be necessary to watch the results and complications of this operation in larger numbers of patients before it can be fully endorsed.

In summary, many surgical procedures are available to the patient suffering from inflammatory bowel disease. These procedures are designed to relieve symptoms, treat life-threatening complications, cure the patient with ulcerative colitis, and greatly improve the quality of life for the patient with Crohn's disease.

9

THE THREAT
OF CANCER

As recently as ten years ago, frank discussion of cancer risks with ulcerative colitis patients was considered taboo by most physicians. The issue was felt to be too "sensitive," and patients would be unduly alarmed. But we have all come a long way since then. Times have changed: doctor-patient relationships have become less authoritarian, as patients' sophistication and demands for their own "right to know" have steadily increased. Today, there is probably not a single reader of this chapter who is not already aware that people with ulcerative colitis stand a significantly higher risk of developing cancer of the colon and rectum than do people without colitis. (Except for cancer of the colon and rectum, there is no evidence that ulcerative colitis patients have higher rates of any other types of cancer than the general population.)

Yet beyond this general awareness of an increased risk of colorectal cancer, there are some questions that require more detailed answers. While these answers are still not fully known nor agreed upon even by experts in the field, this chapter will begin by trying to present as fully as possible our current state of understanding of each of these issues as they relate to cancer in ulcerative colitis. The problems of cancer in Crohn's disease will be discussed later in the chapter.

ULCERATIVE COLITIS

How great is the cancer risk in ulcerative colitis? In other words, what is the actual incidence of colorectal cancer in these patients, and to what extent is this incidence increased over that for people of the same age and sex in the general population?

Even this simplest and most fundamental of questions does not have an easy answer. Different groups of investigators look at the problem from different vantage points. They each see different kinds of patients and often employ different methods of statistical analysis. The complexity of the situation can be measured by the following three considerations.

First of all, the cancer incidence in ulcerative colitis cannot be determined simply by taking the charts of 100 such patients from a doctor's office and counting up how many of them have colorectal cancer in follow-up. Such a crude tally would probably yield only two or three cases of cancer, and would grossly underestimate the risk. There are at least four reasons. For one, some of the patients among the hypothetical hundred would have moved away or become otherwise lost to follow-up. Second, some might presumably have died. Moreover, many would undoubtedly have undergone colectomy and thus could not legitimately be included among the group still at risk for developing colon cancer. Finally, these 100 theoretical patients would all have had colitis for varying lengths of time, so that those who had been sick for only a year or two could not be counted as carrying the same total lifetime risk of cancer development as those who had had colitis for fifteen or twenty years. Statistical steps must be taken, therefore, to correct for these circumstances of patients being followed for varying lengths of time or dropping out of the population at risk. The most common statistical techniques employed for this purpose are called actuarial, or life-table methods. They paint a much more accurate picture of cancer incidence than crude tabulations can achieve.

A second indication of the complexity of the cancer-incidence question is the realization that at any given moment, not every cancer of the colon or rectum has been detected. A short-term survey of cancer incidence among a group of ulcerative colitis patients will again underestimate the risk unless all the patients have had recent barium enemas or colonoscopies. Of course, this detection dilemma becomes minimized as the survey period gets longer, since it is a reasonable assumption that given enough time, all colorectal cancers will unfortunately make their presence known.

The third and perhaps thorniest difficulty in assessing cancer incidence is that the figures will vary drastically depending upon which physician's patients are being studied. No one doctor sees every ulcerative colitis patient in the world, and those patients seen by different doctors have very different clinical characteristics and hence very different probabilities of having cancer. For example, young internists in private practice may have a sense of false security about the colitis-associated cancer issue—either because they haven't been following enough patients long enough to have noticed this outcome, or because when their patients begin experiencing new and worsening symptoms, they take themselves off to other specialists. On the other hand, colorectal surgeons may be inclined to overestimate the cancer incidence, since a disproportionate number of patients might be selectively referred to them for the management of cancers that other doctors have already diagnosed. And by the same token, the worst overestimates of all are liable to be made by the very doctors who publish most of the studies on this subject—namely, surgeons and gastroenterologists at major referral hospitals known for their special interest and expertise in both ulcerative colitis and cancer. Such specialty centers are bound to end up seeing colitis-associated cancer cases far out of proportion to the incidence in otherwise healthy colitis patients who are out walking the streets and not being admitted to famous university hospitals.

So given all these conflicting considerations, what can we conclude about the "true" incidence of cancer in ulcerative colitis? Unless we scrupulously follow many hundreds of colitis patients prospectively from their first date of diagnosis for many decades thereafter, we will never ascertain this elusive "true" incidence. One guess we can make from all the studies available suggests that among ulcerative colitis patients carrying their disease for twenty to thirty years, remaining alive and in follow-up, with their colons still in place, and presenting for one reason or another to major teaching hospitals with special interests in colitis, the total cumulative percentage of such patients who will at some point have developed colorectal cancer lies somewhere in the range of 20 to 30 percent. Considering the relatively small numbers of patients who fit this description in every detail, the absolute number of cancer cases is not very large, but the potential risk is not one to be ignored either.

WHO IS AT RISK?

What clinical characteristics of certain ulcerative colitis patients represent *risk factors* for the development of colorectal cancer? What features identify patients whose risk is highest?

There is much more agreement about risk factors for colitis-associated cancer than there is about precise rates of incidence. There is, for example, universal consensus that the cancer risk rises with increasing duration of inflammatory bowel disease. No evidence for heightened risk can be detected in patients with colitis of less than eight to ten years' duration: the risk appears to rise progressively thereafter. Similarly, there is general agreement that cancer risk is significantly greater when ulcerative colitis involves the entire colon as opposed to only a part of the colon. Patients with only the lower one-third to one-half of the large intestine affected by colitis still seem to have a measurably higher cancer risk than the general population, but it may take about ten years longer for this risk to be manifested than in patients with total colon involvement ("universal" or "pan-" colitis). In cases of simple proctitis or proctosigmoiditis, on the other hand, no increased cancer risk has been statistically detectable.

It once was believed that patients who developed ulcerative colitis in childhood bore an inherently higher cancer risk than patients whose colitis appeared later in life. Several studies have now shown, however, that childhood onset of colitis carries no higher risk of cancer than adult onset, given the same total duration and anatomical extent of disease.

Likewise, there used to be an impression that cancer risk was higher in cases of colitis that had a particularly severe onset or a persistently active clinical course. Once again, current evidence does not support this point of view. Longstanding, clinically quiescent disease appears to carry at least as high a risk as cases that have been chronically symptomatic over the years.

In summary, then, total duration and anatomical extent of disease are the only two factors that have been clearly shown to influence the incidence of colorectal cancer in patients with ulcerative colitis.

WHAT IS THE NATURAL HISTORY OF COLITIS-ASSOCIATED CANCER?

Most cancers of the colon in the general population are thought to arise initially from benign polyps. In ulcerative colitis, on the other hand, cancer seems to develop directly from the mucosa, or surface lining, of the bowel wall itself, without passing through any preliminary benign polypoid stage. Colitis-associated cancers also tend to appear concurrently in multiple locations within the colon approximately four times more commonly than do ordinary colorectal cancers (12 percent versus 3 percent, respectively). Cancers in ulcerative colitis patients, moreover, have an unusual propensity to infiltrate extensive lengths of bowel wall, instead of concentrating in localized sites as most colon cancers do.

Another hallmark of colorectal cancer in ulcerative colitis is that it occurs in patients who are much younger on the average than are those who develop colorectal cancer in the absence of colitis. While the mean age for development of carcinoma of the colon in the general population is in the range of 60, among patients with ulcerative colitis it is 38 years old. Roughly one-third of colitis patients with colorectal cancer develop this malignancy between the ages of 20 and 45.

For all these reasons, the conclusion is inescapable that colorectal cancer is more common in patients with ulcerative colitis, and that its biological behavior is distinctly different.

WHAT IS THE PROGNOSIS OF COLITIS-ASSOCIATED CANCER?

By the time of diagnosis, about half the colorectal cancer in ulcerative colitis patients have already reached an advanced stage. The mortality rate in this group is therefore very high. Most of the unfortunate patients are dead within eighteen months of diagnosis of their cancers. But the other half of the patients, whose cancers are detected in an early stage, do very well and are usually permanently cured after total proctocolectomy and ileostomy. Consequently, the overall survival of ulcerative colitis patients with colorectal cancer is not particularly different from the survival of colorectal cancer patients in the general noncolitis population. The most important practical implication of this fact is that early detection is critical because it saves lives.

HOW CAN COLORECTAL CANCER BE PREVENTED?

The prevention of colitis-associated colorectal cancer is ridiculously easy. Of course, if all colitis patients would undergo total colectomy, then cancer of the colon would be totally prevented in this group. But this extreme solution is hardly practical or desirable. A more useful approach to the cancer problem is to achieve early detection by surveillance of the highest-risk population—namely, patients with more than eight years of total ulcerative colitis or more than fifteen years of left-sided colon disease.

The crucial question, however, is how to survey this population. Thre is no simple blood test or stool examination that has proven useful for cancer screening. The CEA (carcinoembryonic antigen) is not helpful as a screening test either in the general population or among colitis patients. Stool examinations for occult blood (Hemoccult and others),

103

or cytological studies of colon washings are also not totally reliable for detecting early warning signs of cancer in ulcerative colitis. In skillful hands, barium enema examinations can certainly detect cancer of the colon, but by the time colitis-associated cancers have grown big enough to be seen on X rays, it might be too late for cure.

Perhaps the most promising surveillance technique is a combination of sigmoidoscopy with biopsy and colonoscopy with multiple biopsy samplings throughout the colon. There is widespread evidence that certain cellular changes on these biopsies (cellular "dysplasia") herald a significantly increased likelihood that cancer is lurking, or at least on the verge of developing, somewhere within the colon. Not all pathologists agree on the precise criteria for diagnosis of dysplasia, nor is the link between dysplasia and cancer anywhere near a 100 percent phenomenon. Many patients with dysplasia do not have any detectable cancer, and some patients with cancer do not have obvious dysplasia. But we are not talking about certainties, we are talking about probabilities. And in terms of probabilities, the fact remains that there is a much higher risk of cancer in a colon with dysplasia than in a colon without it.

If the dysplasia is far advanced and associated with a mass lesion visible through the colonoscope, the likelihood of malignancy is even greater. In these circumstances, the malignancy may already have passed beyond an easily curable stage. If, on the other hand, dysplasia turns up in biopsies from areas that appear normal to the naked eye, the probability of an associated cancer is somewhat lower, but any such cancers are more likely to be in an earlier stage and therefore curable.

Nobody knows how often colonoscopy and biopsy should be carried out for the most efficient surveillance program in high-risk colitis patients. The most often recommended schedule in our current limited stage of knowledge is every year or two. There is even less consensus among experts as to whether or not the finding of dysplasia is an absolute indication for colectomy in order to avoid further cancer risk. Many doctors believe it is such an indication; but even those who do not, agree that finding dysplasia is cause for extremely vigilant follow-up.

Whatever practice a physician chooses to adopt, the age is long past when important medical and surgical decisions can be made without input from patients. The burden of decision making concerning surveillance programs and colectomies should not be shifted onto them, but patients must be adequately informed of pros and cons, of risks and benefits, so that their own needs and wishes can be weighed heavily in the balance. For many patients, the choice is made easier by the assurance that total colectomy cures ulcerative colitis, and that several new surgical alternatives to standard ileostomy have been developed.

CROHN'S DISEASE

As in ulcerative colitis, patients with Crohn's disease have no significantly increased risk of cancer outside the gastrointestinal tract. But even if we restrict our attention to gastrointestinal cancer, we have to look beyond the colon and rectum, since Crohn's disease usually involves the small intestine as well.

As far as colorectal cancer is concerned, there is steadily mounting evidence that the incidence might be measurably higher in patients with Crohn's colitis than in the general population. The magnitude of this increased risk is not as great as for ulcerative colitis. The increased cancer risk in Crohn's colitis has been calculated as being approximately one-third that in universal ulcerative colitis. On the other hand, Crohn's disease rarely affects the entire colon; partial or segmental involvement is the usual rule. A more appropriate comparison, therefore, might be between Crohn's colitis and partial or left-sided ulcerative colitis. By this standard, the cancer risks in the two diseases are more nearly comparable, and the need for surveillance would be about the same. This was the conclusion of a recent NFIC study of cancer incidence in Crohn's disease.

Also, more people with Crohn's disease will have had surgery, and will not have carried disease in their colons for as long as people with ulcerative colitis. It is therefore not yet possible to know whether cases of Crohn's disease and ulcerative colitis of the same extent and duration may ultimately turn out to hold comparable cancer risks.

With respect to cancer of the small intestine, there is absolutely no doubt that the incidence is relatively increased in cases of Crohn's disease as compared to the general population. In fact, the overall rate of small bowel cancer in Crohn's disease patients is more than 100 times greater than the expected rate in normal people of the same age and sex. But small bowel cancer is one of the rarest of all malignancies to begin with. To say that its incidence is relatively increased in Crohn's disease is still to say that it is an extremely uncommon occurrence. Indeed, there are scarcely more than fifty such cases ever recorded in the entire world's literature on Crohn's disease, so this is hardly a worry that should keep anyone lying awake at night.

The risk of small bowel cancer does not even begin to appear until after two or three decades of Crohn's disease. Most patients have had their segments of diseased bowel surgically removed before that time. Only those few surgical patients who have had their affected areas bypassed instead of resected continue to run any measurable cancer risk postoperatively. About 40 percent of all reported cases of small bowel cancer in Crohn's disease have occurred in bypassed loops. For this reason, surgeons today prefer, whenever possible, to remove rather than bypass sections of diseased intestine.

PART III
Living with the Diseases

10

CROHN'S DISEASE AND ULCERATIVE COLITIS IN CHILDREN

During the last decade, there has been an increasing awareness that Crohn's disease and ulcerative colitis affect children. In one large study, 20 percent of adult patients with Crohn's disease exhibited some signs of the illness before age 15. A smaller percentage of patients with ulcerative colitis showed symptoms as children. In general, these conditions are rarely diagnosed in infancy, but begin to be recognized at 5 to 7 years of age and especially between the ages of 10 and 18. About 25 percent of these children have a family member with Crohn's disease or ulcerative colitis. However, for the majority of children, there is no known family history of either of these conditions. The diagnosis thus becomes the first step in the process of learning about inflammatory bowel disease.

EARLY SIGNS AND SYMPTOMS

While many of the symptoms are similar in children and

adults, certain features are of particular importance to pediatric patients. At times, the early signs (fatigue, low-grade fever, decreased appetite, vague abdominal pain) are subtle. This often results in a delay in the recognition, diagnosis, and treatment of these conditions. It is not unusual for the symptoms to be attributed to school difficulties, "laziness," or emotional problems. Eventually, the persistence of these signs leads to the correct diagnosis.

In general, symptoms correspond to the area of the intestine which is most inflamed (Table 2). Children with ulcerative colitis usually have cramping followed by bloody diarrhea. The pain often diminishes after the bowel movements occur. Crohn's disease of the small intestine frequently is associated with pain in the periumbilical (navel) area, especially after meals. When the colon is involved, diarrhea is common. Weight loss occurs in both conditions but tends to be greater in Crohn's disease because of the longer duration of disease prior to diagnosis.

Table 2: PERCENTAGE OF CHILDREN WITH IBD SHOWING SIGNS AND SYMPTOMS

	Crohn's Disease (52 patients)	Ulcerative Colitis (22 patients)
Abdominal Pain	88%	95%
Change in Stool Pattern	81%	91%
Blood in Stool	54%	100%
Weight Loss	87%	68%
Fever	54%	41%
Decrease in Height Percentile	36%	14%

Since the extent and severity of the intestinal involvement is variable, discussions between the child, the parent, and the physician should encourage questioning and an exchange of information. Diagrams are often extremely helpful. They enable children to understand why their cooperation in taking medications helps to control disease activity.

THE PROBLEM OF POOR GROWTH

Interference with growth is one of the unique aspects of childhood inflammatory bowel disease. Many people, including some physicians, think that this poor growth is caused only by cortiscosteroids such as prednisone or ACTH. It is now recognized that a slowing in the growth rate may occur before any treatment begins. Impaired growth can be documented by plotting the child's height on standard growth curves (see Figure 11). These charts are usually available from a pediatrician or family physician, and parents are strongly urged to use them to keep track of their child's growth pattern. Most children tend to follow their own curve or "height percentile" on these charts. When a child grows less than two inches per year or falls onto a lower curve, the situation should be discussed with the child's physician. Growth is most affected when children have a prolonged bout of active disease during periods of normally rapid growth such as the adolescent growth spurt.

The cause of the growth failure in inflammatory bowel disease is under active investigation. It was initially thought that growth hormone levels were lower than normal in children with IBD. One small group of children with IBD received growth hormone therapy, but no significant increase in the growth rate occurred. It is now recognized that growth hormone levels are normal, and in fact, may be higher than normal in children with these diseases. Thyroid function tests are also normal. Therefore replacement therapy with either of these hormones is not used for growth-

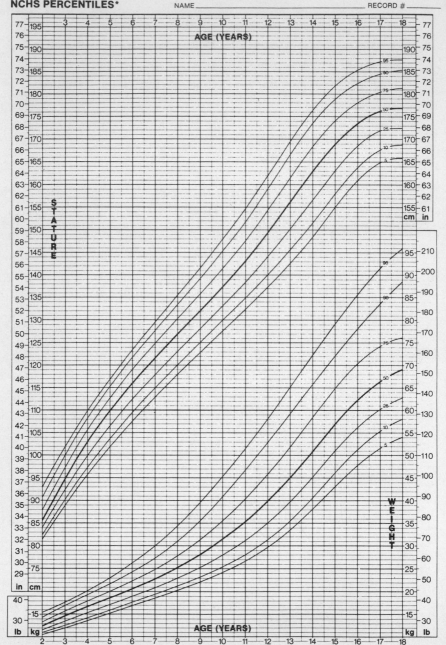

Figure 11A. Boys 2-18 yrs.: Normal growth curves for children and adolescents, Data from the National Center for Health Statistics, Hyattsville, Maryland.

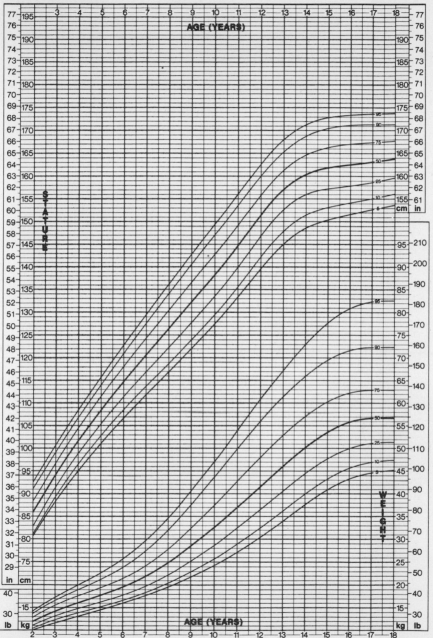

Figure 11B. Girls 2-18 yrs.: Normal growth curves for children and adolescents, Data from the National Center for Health Statistics, Hyattsville, Maryland.

impaired children with inflammatory bowel disease.

Poor absorption of nutrients is a potential cause of growth failure. This situation develops in children with extensive small bowel disease or after resections of large areas of intestine. However, most children with growth failure do not have significant malabsorption. The major problem is a decreased intake of food. This is the result, at least in part, of abdominal cramping, and is manifested in changes in stool pattern which follow eating.

ADEQUATE CALORIC INTAKE ESSENTIAL FOR GROWTH IN IBD

Studies of the nutritional effects of inflammatory bowel disease in childhood have contributed to our understanding of growth failure. Initially, weight gain and increased growth were observed following the intravenous administration of nutrients. Subsequently, improved growth was reported in children with Crohn's disease who were given supplemental formulas orally. These results are explained by recent studies which show that growth-impaired children eat only one-half the calories recommended for their age group. It is now believed that careful attention to nutrient intake, particularly calories and protein, is important in reducing the likelihood of growth impairment. Nutritional goals should therefore be part of the therapeutic plan. Caloric intakes in the range of 75 to 80 calories per kilogram body weight, which meet the Recommended Dietary Allowance (RDA) for age, usually improve growth in children with growth failure. Protein intakes of approximately 1.5 to 2.0 grams per kilogram body weight are also recommended. If milk products produce gastrointestinal discomfort or increase symptoms, the child should be tested for lactose intolerance. Commerical products are available that degrade lactose into simple sugars (e.g. Lact-Aid®).

The method used to provide nutritional support depends entirely upon the activity and severity of the intestinal symptoms. Whenever possible, the oral route is used. At times, nutrients must be given intravenously. It is important to emphasize that control of symptoms is necessary before the child or teenager can consume an adequate dietary intake. As the course of the illness fluctuates, changes in medications may be necessary. The mechanisms by which nutritional support improves growth are now better understood, so certain deficiencies can be corrected and energy needs met. Several research projects are under way in which investigators are seeking to understand this problem more completely.

Continuing disease activity may also cause a slowing in the rate of sexual maturation. Adolescents may show delayed development of the physical signs of maturation, including late menstruation in girls. Similarly, temporary cessation of menses may follow a significant weight loss in girls who have previously had menstrual periods. Control of the disease activity and appropriate weight gain usually result in resumption of normal sexual development. Attention to these aspects of the adolescent's overall well-being is extremely important. When there are problems or concerns, the child or teenager should be encouraged to discuss these openly with the physician.

JOINT PAINS IN CHILDREN

Painful joints are another frequent systemic manifestation of inflammatory bowel disease in children (see Chapter 5). In fact, it has been estimated that at least 25 percent of children will have arthralgia (painful or stiff joints) or arthritis (swollen warm joints). Usually the knees, ankles, or hips are affected. Frequently, the joint pain will subside when the activity of the intestinal disease decreases. On occasion, joint symptoms may begin before intestinal complaints occur. This causes some patients to be incorrectly diagnosed as having juvenile rheumatoid arthritis rather than inflammatory bowel disease. At times, medications that relieve joint pain are indicated. It is reassuring to know that unlike other forms of arthritis, involvement of the joints in IBD does not lead to permanent changes or deformity. There is, however, one unusual form of arthritis which does cause permanent changes in the spine. Fortunately this form is rare, and is not related to IBD.

Children and teenagers sometimes have difficulty understanding why doctors ask detailed questions regarding abdominal cramping, characteristics of bowel movements, menstrual periods, etc. This information provides clues so that the physician can select the most appropriate medications to control the disease activity.

When the disease is most active, it may be necessary to alter school responsibilities, and to limit participation in sports. The student should become familiar with the location of all the bathroom facilities in school. Parents may need to request permission for children to leave the classroom discreetly. Regular school attendance should be encouraged except when symptoms require additional rest or intensive medical management. It is not at all unusual for the young person to feel disappointed, angry, or depressed when the disease becomes active. It takes a continuing cooperative effort by the patient, family, and physician to find a plan of therapy which diminishes the intestinal symptoms and promotes a sense of well-being.

DIAGNOSTIC TESTS

Several factors will help the physician decide which medication to prescribe. The intensity of symptoms (fever, cramping, and stool frequency) is important. At times, laboratory tests provide additional useful information. Those that are particularly helpful in childhood inflammatory bowel disease are:

- the blood count (hemoglobin/hematocrit)—to determine if anemia is present
- sedimentation rate—may reflect the degree of inflammation
- serum protein levels (including albumin)—may indicate degree of malnutrition
- mineral levels—e.g. iron
- vitamins—folic acid, vitamin B-12

Sometimes, direct observation of the appearance of the intestinal lining is necessary to assess the severity of the inflammation. While these tests are not pleasant, they are frequently the only way to evaluate the activity of the disease. Children usually cooperate with the physician in performing an endoscopy if the procedure is explained fully and the child's trust is obtained. X rays of the intestine are always a part of the initial evaluation, unless the disease is too severe. From time to time, blood tests and X-ray examinations may need to be repeated.

MEDICATIONS FOR IBD

Sulfasalazine (Azulfidine) and cortiscosteroids (prednisone, methylprednisolone, hydrocortisone, etc.) are the most frequently prescribed medications for both Crohn's disease and ulcerative colitis. In some instances, other antibiotics or medications that suppress inflammation may be prescribed. It should be emphasized that the administration of cortiscosteroids to children and teenagers must be managed carefully to avoid growth suppression. Therefore, in this age group, daily cortiscosteroids are given only when necessary to control active disease. They may be gradually decreased to an every-other-day schedule for some patients. Once the disease is controlled, children and teenagers usually grow normally and may even increase their growth rate above normal, achieving "catch-up growth."

WHEN SURGERY MAY BE NEEDED

The indications for surgery in children with inflammatory bowel disease are in many ways similar to those of adults. When impaired growth is recognized and nutritional support is not helpful, surgical intervention may be indicated, especially if the child has not yet reached puberty. Operations performed during later stages of puberty and beyond may not allow an adequate period of time for accelerated and significant growth to occur. If there are no complications from Crohn's disease, however, intestinal resections are best not performed because of the very high risk of the disease recurring.

It is important to emphasize that children and teenagers with inflammatory bowel disease should be encouraged to discuss their symptoms and feelings with their family and physician. Continuing support from the physician is essential in helping the child learn how to cope with the fluctuations in disease activity. Parents are encouraged to understand as much as possible about the disease and its emotional effects and to try to encourage independence in the child. Family therapy and mutual help groups may provide strong psychological support for the ill child and the family (Figure 12).

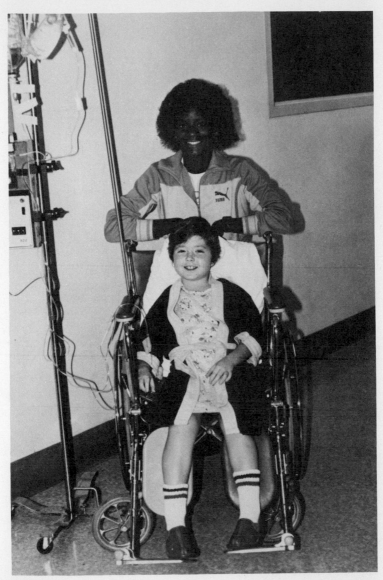

Figure 12. Track star and Olympic hopeful Rene Felton visits a young Crohn's disease patient at the U.C.L.A. Medical Center. Rene herself has suffered from Crohn's disease since the age of 11.

11

PREGNANCY

Both Crohn's disease and ulcerative colitis are primarily diseases of young people. Since females are as likely to be affected as males, it is important to know how pregnancy will influence the course of disease, and how the diseases will affect the outcome of pregnancy. The material in this chapter is based on recent studies, including a national survey involving a large number of pregnant women with IBD.

The first thing most women with IBD want to know is whether they will be able to conceive as easily as other women. Those women who have had difficulty conceiving have usually had Crohn's disease (often with disease in the colon), and not ulcerative colitis. This lack of fertility is usually temporary, and probably is not caused by any mechanical blocking of the Fallopian tubes. It is probably caused by the symptoms of active Crohn's disease—fever, fistulas, and anemia. If a woman with Crohn's disease has difficulty conceiving, she may need more vigorous treatment of her disease. In this case, it may be a good idea to postpone pregnancy until the symptoms are under control, and the woman feels stronger.

While being pregnant will not harm a woman with Crohn's disease or ulcerative colitis, any woman contemplating pregnancy should consider the state of her health before conceiving. According to recent studies, women with either illness should do well during the pregnancy if disease was inactive at the time of conception. However, if a pregnancy occurs during a period of active disease, either disease is likely to remain active or to worsen. This worsening generally occurs during the first trimester (three months) in ulcerative colitis and the third trimester in Crohn's disease. If either disease can be brought into remission with drug therapy during the pregnancy, the woman's health should be good for the remainder of the pregnancy.

Most pregnant women with IBD have normal deliveries and healthy babies in roughly the same proportions as healthy women in the general population. If there is a problem affecting the pregnancy, it generally occurs in women with active Crohn's disease. These women run a greater risk of premature delivery, stillbirth, or spontaneous abortion. If the symptoms become severe enough to require surgery, the risk to the fetus becomes even greater.

It is not unknown for IBD to have its onset during pregnancy. There are many reports of ulcerative colitis starting during pregnancy, but recent studies have shown that such incidence is no more severe than at any other time. Crohn's disease may also begin during pregnancy, and both diseases may begin during the postpartum period (the weeks immediately following delivery), but this is very rare.

TAKING MEDICATION DURING PREGNANCY

It is only natural for the pregnant woman and her obstetrician to want to restrict all medications during pregnancy to avoid possible harm to the fetus. Sulfasalazine and prednisone are the two drugs used most commonly to control the symptoms of Crohn's disease and ulcerative colitis. A recent national study has found no evidence that the fetus is harmed by either of these drugs taken by the mother during pregnancy.

Since the major threat to the pregnancy appears to come from the active disease itself and not from the medication, these drugs should not be discontinued when a woman becomes pregnant. If either disease worsens severely during the pregnancy, prednisone and/or sulfasalazine may be introduced or increased. Sulfasalazine may also be used to maintain a remission for the remainder of the pregnancy and after.

The side effects of these medications are generally no greater when they are taken during pregnancy. However, sulfasalazine may cause nausea which compounds that commonly experienced in early pregnancy. The drug may also aggravate the heartburn sometimes experienced in the later months of pregnancy. If this happens, it might be helpful to switch to enteric-coated sulfasalazine tablets.

Many women taking sulfasalazine or prednisone want to know if they can nurse their babies. Although some sulfasalazine does pass into the breast milk, its concentration is much reduced, and to our knowledge, it has not been shown to harm the newborn. The dosage of prednisone should be reduced and the drug discontinued as quickly as possible in any patient, whether pregnant or not. If a new mother wishes to nurse her baby while still taking a moderate or high dose of prednisone, the baby's health should be monitored carefully by the pediatrician.

Physicians are much more cautious about using immunosuppressive drugs such as azathioprine and 6-mercaptopurine during pregnancy. Animal studies using these drugs have found evidence of genetic damage to offspring. At present, there are no studies of the genetic effects of these drugs in humans. Since our experience with immunosuppressives is so limited, patients are advised *not* to become pregnant while taking these drugs. If conception does occur while a woman is taking these medications, therapeutic abortion may be advisable. (In the past, a severe flare-up of ulcerative colitis was occasionally treated by therapeutic abortion. The results were mixed: the disease improved in some patients but not in others. Today, therapeutic abortion is rarely, if ever, performed for this reason. Instead, the patient is treated vigorously with drug therapy in an effort to control symptoms.)

There is no reason why a sigmoidoscopy, rectal biopsy, or gastroscopy cannot be performed on the pregnant patient if these tests are necessary in the management of the disease. A limited colonoscopy with flexible colonoscope may also be performed, if necessary. Diagnostic X rays should be postponed until after delivery.

SURGERY AND PREGNANCY

Whenever possible, surgery for Crohn's disease or ulcerative colitis should be postponed until after delivery. However, if the disease is severe and not responding to drug therapy, it may be more dangerous to the patient not to operate. It is a matter of weighing the risks. Although there are reports of intestinal resections and even of ileostomies performed successfully in pregnant women, when any abdominal surgery is performed, the likelihood that the fetus will survive is reduced.

Many women worry that previous bowel surgery might affect the course of their pregnancy. In Crohn's disease, previous bowel resection does not appear to affect the pregnancy in any way. In fact, since resection usually results in remission of symptoms, the patient is likely to have an easier pregnancy than she would have with active disease.

Women with ileostomies for ulcerative colitis (or sometimes for Crohn's disease) occasionally suffer prolapse or obstruction of the ileostomy during pregnancy. It is best to postpone pregnancy for one year after the ileostomy is constructed (whether conventional or continent ileostomy) to allow the body time to adapt to it. In Crohn's disease complicated by abcesses or fistulas around the rectum, episiotomy (standard surgery to widen the birth canal) may have to be avoided. In these cases, delivery is by Cesarean section.

DIET AND STRESS DURING PREGNANCY

In general, the pregnant woman with Crohn's disease or ulcerative colitis should follow the same well-balanced diet recommended for all pregnant women. The obstetrician and/or gastroenterologist may recommend the addition of specific foods, vitamins, and minerals.

If the disease is active, however, it may be necessary to eliminate foods from the diet which cause discomfort. The NFIC brochure *Questions and Answers about Diet and Nutrition in Ileitis and Colitis* contains helpful advice on such foods.

Emotional stress may cause symptoms to worsen during pregnancy, just as it may at any other time. But this does not mean that stress plays any role in causing the disease. Similarly, the postpartum period is a time normally characterized by rapid change, both physical and emotional, in the new mother. These changes may also cause a temporary worsening of symptoms. For this reason it is a good idea to keep in close touch with your gastroenterologist during the postpartum period.

12

CROHN'S DISEASE AND ULCERATIVE COLITIS IN OLDER PEOPLE

Inflammatory bowel disease is commonly thought of as a disorder of the younger years. A worried parent or a young adult fearing that the most active period of life will be hampered by this disease are the images that frequently come to mind when IBD is mentioned. Unfortunately, with certain exceptions, IBD has little respect for age. This chapter will deal with the patient with previously documented IBD who is approaching later life, and with the older patient who becomes ill with IBD for the first time in the later years.

OLD DISEASE IN THE OLDER PATIENT

Many patients who experience the onset of IBD earlier in life are understandably concerned about how the course of disease will vary as they approach their later years. Will it become quiescent? Will surgery become necessary? How will they manage their attacks when they are older? Will the attacks become more severe? Little information is available on these subjects. Every gastroenterologist and surgeon is familiar with patients whose disease appears to "burn out" in the later years; attacks become less frequent and sometimes disappear completely. This is the situation for which patient and physician alike hope will occur.

For those patients whose disease remains active into the later years, several factors need to be considered. These include the risk of carcinoma, the increased mortality and morbidity with severe attacks, and problems associated with advancing age.

The risk of cancer in IBD was discussed in Chapter 9. As noted previously, since cancer in ulcerative colitis is related to duration of disease, it is not surprising that patients who develop this complication are more likely to have had the disease for several decades and to be in a relatively older age group. Thus the older patient with active ulcerative colitis who has had the disease for several decades represents a group with a particularly high risk and a need for vigilant surveillance. In contrast, patients who first develop ulcerative colitis in the later years bear a smaller risk of cancer.

Fulminant attacks of IBD may cause a particularly high mortality rate in older patients. For this reason, many physicians feel that an aggressive (surgical) approach is warranted earlier in patients failing to respond to medical management. Despite their fears about learning to care for an ileostomy, most of these patients learn quickly. Elderly patients with a diminished capacity to heal, many of whom are on long-term steroid therapy, constitute a group that can be expected to have increased mortality if surgery is unduly postponed. Most patients beyond the age of 60, however, will still respond favorably to medical treatment.

NEW DISEASE IN THE OLDER PATIENT:
IS IT IBD?

Physicians have known for some time that inflammatory bowel disease (ulcerative colitis much more than Crohn's disease) seems to show a second peak of attack in older Americans between the ages of 50 and 70. The number of patients who become ill with IBD later in life, however, is much smaller than the number who are stricken in their teens and twenties.

Recent reappraisal of cases of IBD diagnosed in later life has yielded some interesting new information. In the last twenty years, gastroenterologists and surgeons have learned that the bowel, particularly the colon, is subject to a form of ulcerating disease that develops with age because of inadequate blood supply (ischemia). This "ischemic" colitis, primarily a disease of later life (as are circulatory diseases such as coronary artery disease and poor circulation in the legs), may mimic such symptoms of IBD as diarrhea, blood in the stools, and abdominal pain. In a recent review of eighty-one patients whose symptoms of colitis began after the age of 50, three-quarters of them actually had ischemic colitis, not IBD. Furthermore, a third of these ischemic colitis patients had been misdiagnosed originally as having ulcerative colitis or Crohn's disease. For this reason, special care must be taken to differentiate IBD from other inflammatory intestinal conditions that occur in the older patient. Sometimes, only observation over weeks or months will clarify the picture.

Antibiotic-associated colitis, discussed earlier, is another recently described form of colitis that seems to occur with increased frequency or ferocity in the elderly patient. This colitis is caused by toxins produced by bacteria that are given a selective advantage for growth in the colon because of the administration of certain antibiotics. Symptoms of this type of colitis may be quite prolonged and therefore may mimic the symptoms of IBD.

Diverticular disease of the colon also may complicate diagnosis in this age group. Diverticula are small sacs that protrude from the lining of the colon into and through the wall of this organ and may perforate it, causing pain, fever, and bleeding. Diverticula may cause inflammation resembling the segmental inflammation characteristic of Crohn's colitis. These diverticula may also lead to fistulas within the wall of the bowel, to other organs (urinary bladder), or even to the skin itself, again closely imitating some features of Crohn's disease.

There are also infectious conditions that closely simulate IBD. For example, infection with campylobacter bacteria may mimic ulcerative colitis. It was probably campylobacter colitis misdiagnosed as "atypical" ulcerative colitis in the past when physicians were unable to culture this bacteria from the stool.

NEW IBD IN THE OLDER PATIENT: HOW DOES IT BEHAVE?

As has been indicated, although it is rarer than previously believed, IBD does occur in elderly patients. Is there a predictable difference in the course of the disease when the onset occurs in later life?

In the reappraisal of colitis in the elderly mentioned above, only eleven patients with newly diagnosed ulcerative colitis were found in the group of eighty-one patients. Although the course of their disease was variable (as is the course of any group of patients with ulcerative colitis), it was somewhat more severe than that seen in younger patients with the same disease. Surgery was more often necessary than might have been predicted in younger patients. The disease was more often associated with complications outside the intestinal tract such as arthritis, skin rash, or inflammation of the eyes.

Crohn's disease in the older individual seems predominantly to affect women. Furthermore, it seems to run a more compressed and severe course when it occurs in the elderly patient. Among thirty-three patients from one Boston hospital with onset of Crohn's disease after age 60, more than one-half required surgery; in the study described above, *all* patients with late onset of Crohn's disease required surgery.

This severity of late-onset IBD may be caused by the frequent concomitants of aging rather than by the disease. For example, the anemia that so often accompanies IBD may be well tolerated by the young adult who has no other medical problems. It is far more dangerous in the older patient with other common medical problems associated with aging, such as coronary artery disease. Similarly, corticosteroids that are useful in many cases of IBD, tend to complicate and worsen diabetes, osteoporosis (bone resorption), hypertension, and other diseases that are age-related. Patients with these problems are often referred to surgery earlier in the course of their disease specifically to avoid complicating one disease with the added presence of another.

It is generally believed that older patients have a lowered resistance to disease in general, attributed to waning competence of the immunologic systems which protect us all, and to slowing of the reparative processes that restore damaged tissue. Any or all of these factors may explain why surgery seems necessary more often in the older patient who first develops IBD, and why the disease appears to run a more severe course.

We have come a long way in our understanding of inflamatory bowel disease in the older population. As our knowledge deepens and expands through basic research into the mechanisms of disease, our therapeutic skills will no doubt improve as well.

13

THE ROLE OF
THE EMOTIONS

For years, people with Crohn's disease and ulcerative colitis have been in doubt about the nature of the relationship between the disease and their emotions. In addition to coping with a difficult and unpredictable illness, an illness that leaves no part of their lives untouched, many of these people have also been labeled with a wide variety of psychiatric diagnoses. Patients and their families have experienced much unnecessary guilt and anxiety because of the myth that Crohn's disease and ulcerative colitis are "psychosomatic" diseases. They have had to live with the misconception, long held by uninformed physicians and by the public, that the pain and diarrhea of IBD can be "turned off" if the patient becomes less anxious, less focused on his or her body. To complicate matters further, Crohn's disease and ulcerative colitis are often confused with the misnomer "spastic colitis" (irritable bowel syndrome), a far less serious condition that may indeed have a relationship to the emotions, but has little in common with inflammatory bowel disease.

EARLY PSYCHOANALYTIC STUDIES

What exactly is the role of emotional factors in inflammatory bowel disease? In the past, psychiatrists considered these diseases to be psychosomatic, partly because the nervous system profoundly affects bowel function, and partly because the origin of the diseases could not be explained in any other way. These psychiatrists analyzed small groups of IBD patients in the hospital, and found some common symptoms and traits which they called the colitis personality. The patients they studied were found to be compulsive, conformist, overly dependent, passive, and unable to express anger. Other studies found a connection between the death of a parent or spouse or other severe emotional stress, and the onset of Crohn's disease or ulcerative colitis. Several early studies branded the mothers of patients as domineering and overprotective.

The trouble with these early studies was that they focused on chronically sick IBD patients, people whose lives had been interrupted by repeated bouts with illness. Very few of these studies used people with other chronic illnesses or healthy people as control groups. Many researchers began to question whether studying sick patients in a hospital environment without proper controls was a valid way to determine what role emotional factors might play in the disease process.

CHRONIC ILLNESS AS A CAUSE OF STRESS

Recent studies of the relationship between emotional factors and the inflammatory bowel diseases have attempted to correct the flaws in the methods used in past studies. They have used both hospitalized patients and healthy people as controls, and these controls are usually matched to the IBD group for age and sex. These newer studies have generally failed to find evidence of significant emotional illness or disability in groups of IBD patients. While there is little doubt that emotional stress can stimulate or aggravate physical symptoms like diarrhea and abdominal pain, most physicians who treat inflammatory bowel disease no longer feel that stress plays any role in causing the diseases. Rather, they emphasize the emotional impact of the disease on patients, and the difficulties encountered in coping with symptoms. They seem to understand that when individuals must endure frequent attacks of pain, bleeding, and many trips to the bathroom, it is very difficult for them to conduct their lives as before. In fact, one recent study showed that depression was the most common psychiatric symptom found in a group of IBD patients. Most physicians who treat these patients now view these depressions as a reaction to the stress and disruptions in living imposed by chronic inflammatory bowel disease.

Treatments and medication, too, may impose a stressful burden of their own. Diagnostic tests that must be repeated periodically, such as the upper GI series, barium enema, colonoscopy, or sigmoidoscopy, can be embarrassing and even humiliating for some patients. The need to take medications with many side effects—some of them temporarily disfiguring—may cause feelings of depression. This is particularly true of the corticosteroids (prednisone, hydrocortisone, etc.). According to Drs. M. J. Goodman and M. Sparberg,

Steroids can also have effects on the mood of the patient. They can lead to depression, or mania, or to a sense of euphoria; and sleeplessness can be a side effect. . . . The patient's appetite can increase. This can be useful in some nutritionally depleted patients. . . but some patients become excessively obese.

THE NEED FOR SUPPORT

With the understanding that chronic IBD can create an emotional burden for those afflicted, the physician caring for a person with Crohn's disease or ulcerative colitis should be as patient and understanding as possible. He or she should be able to recognize when the anxiety and depression brought on by the illness is reaching a serious level, severely altering the quality of life. The physician can then suggest and encourage the use of a psychotherapist or family therapist. Many patients cope more successfully with their condition when they have the opportunity to discuss feelings about being chronically ill with understanding professionals.

THE FAMILY: A NEGLECTED RESOURCE

The people closest to the IBD patient—the family—are often the ones who have the most difficulty coming to terms with the illness. Parents may wish to deny the seriousness of a child's disease, due possibly to misplaced guilt, hoping that the child will "outgrow" it. Then they may become depressed at having to accept the reality of chronic pain and illness in a formerly healthy son or daughter. Siblings of a child with Crohn's disease or ulcerative colitis may resent the amount of time and attention spent on the child who is ill. The spouse of an IBD patient may react to the illness by becoming frightened, overprotective, jealous, resentful, angry, or all of these together. The healthy spouse may no longer find the ill spouse sexually attractive. Some family members may not know how to react to the illness, and other relatives may simply ignore it altogether.

Thankfully, there is renewed interest today in helping families of chronically ill persons to function as true support systems for the patient and for each other. Family therapists are professionals who consider that when there is serious chronic illness in one family member, this may disrupt the normal dynamics of family life. These professionals can help family members to sort out and express their feelings about the illness to one another. Through regular meetings with the family, they can help them to express love and support for the sick member and to cope with the episodes of illness and with the emotional hardships imposed by chronic inflammatory bowel disease.

MUTUAL HELP:
AN IDEA WHOSE TIME HAS COME

Sometimes it simply isn't enough to have an understanding and supportive family. It may be of tremendous benefit to meet and talk with other people suffering from the same illness. For many patients, the Mutual Help, Self Help, or other support groups sponsored by NFIC chapters in various cities have provided their first encounter with anyone else with Crohn's disease or ulcerative colitis. These IBD sufferers have reported a great sense of relief at being encouraged to talk about their problems without embarrassment in the presence of people who really care .

For example, since 1980, NFIC's Greater New York Chapter has sponsored a popular series of these Mutual Help groups. Participants meet informally once a week for eight weeks. Group members have included patients, their spouses, and parents of patients in varying combinations. Group leaders are not professionals, but are interested members who have participated in previous groups. Topics for discussion usually include coping with symptoms, coming to terms with the illness, communicating with doctors, family members, and employers, the side effects of medications, and sexual and social problems that may arise. All members of the group are encouraged to relate their experiences and to express themselves. Apart from realizing that they are not alone in their experience with the illness, participants come away with the satisfaction that derives from having helped others.

14

COPING WITH
HOSPITALIZATION

Hospitalization for treatment of Crohn's disease or ulcerative colitis is certainly not something that anyone looks forward to. Hospitals can be impersonal places, and it is all too easy for patients to become discouraged and depressed about being there. It is important to remember, however, that symptoms often improve dramatically during hospitalization and that the inflammation may heal rapidly with appropriate therapy.

The following suggestions are offered in an effort to help you cope with being in the hospital. The basic message is that while there are many people who are doing their very best to help you, there are also many ways in which you can help yourself.

THE ADMISSION PROCEDURE

If you are well enough to walk and to sit for a reasonable

length of time, you should arrange to go directly to the admitting office for admission. Be sure to check your expected time of arrival before leaving for the hospital. If, however, you are feeling weak and experiencing major symptoms, your doctor may advise you to go directly to the hospital's emergency room, where he or she will usually meet you.

Make sure that you have checked whether private as well as semiprivate rooms are available. A private room costs more and may not be covered by your medical insurance policy, but offers the advantages of additional quiet and rest. These are certainly important considerations. Above all, try to secure a hospital room with easy access to a toilet. Even today, there are some hospital rooms that do not have toilet facilities. When you enter the room assigned to you, this is not the time to find out that the nearest toilet is down the corridor!

Bring all your medications with you to the hospital. You may be taking an important and effective medication that cannot be secured by the hospital pharmacy until the next day. For example, there are some forms of rectal steroids that are not stocked in these pharmacies. You should also bring any other items that may be important to you. If a heating pad has been of help at home, you should bring it with you. Before using it, check with your nurse to be absolutely sure that the electric outlet is compatible. If you bring this equipment with you, your treatment can proceed without delay. It is quite likely that the evaluation procedure may take most of the afternoon or evening.

If at all possible, arrange to come to the admitting office *after* lunch and when you reach your room, make sure an evening meal has been ordered for you. If you arrive at the admitting office before lunch and your admission evaluation is delayed until the evening, you could miss both lunch and dinner. If you remind your physician about your dietary needs, he or she can see to it that you receive meals on time.

YOUR HOSPITAL ROOM

In addition to determining whether there is easy access to a bathroom, there are several other aspects of your room that are important. The first is the bed itself. If your buttocks are ulcerated or your perianal tissue very inflamed from diarrhea or perianal disease, you should request either a sheepskin quilt or an air mattress in order to take as much pressure as possible off these sensitive areas.

In addition, if you have difficulty moving from side to side, it is frequently helpful to have an orthopedic frame attached over your bed with a metal triangle that hangs down from the overhead support. By grasping this triangle, you can lift yourself slightly off the bed and make those small adjustments in position that provide comfort.

Decide if you want a telephone. If rest is truly important, you may decide not to activate your telephone when you are sleeping. The same sort of decision can be made regarding a television set.

Above all, determine whether it is possible to turn off the intercom system that permits the hospital page operator to call in all rooms simultaneously looking for a staff person, so it won't disturb your sleep.

THE NURSING STAFF

Your nurses are your best friends while you are in the hospital. Do not hesitate to call on them for assistance, but also remember they are taking care of many other patients, some of whom may have needs that are greater than yours. If you find that they are not responding fast enough or do not appear to be attending to your needs, it is reasonable for you to explain your difficulties in a nice way in an effort to elicit their help. Most nurses will respond positively to this type of interaction. Try to be diplomatic.

Your nurse can be helpful in explaining the preparations for tests, the nature of the tests themselves, and the schedule for your medications. For example, you may find that medications are being given during the middle of the night that could easily be given at bedtime, or given when you awaken rather than at six A.M. The nurse may simply be following the physician's orders to give medicines every six hours. If the order was written at six P.M., your medications must then be given at midnight and again at six A.M. If, on the other hand, the order was transcribed at nine P.M., you may then find your next dosage is at three in the morning! If this happens, it is reasonable to ask the nurse to check with your doctor to see whether your medications can be given on a more reasonable schedule that permits a full night's sleep.

Regarding tests such as X rays, it is important for you to know exactly what preparations you will be receiving. You should already have discussed this with your physician. If you find that a more vigorous preparation is planned than you anticipated—such as different types of enemas and/or cathartics—you should share this concern with your nurse. By assuming responsibility in this way, you can help avoid potential nursing error. Chapter 4 contains a complete description of the kinds of "preps" IBD patients can expect in the hospital.

HOSPITAL DIETICIANS

Since good nutrition is so important to your total recovery, it is helpful to develop a good working relationship with the dietician. Keep accurate notes of what you eat. Arrange for extra snacks and bedtime feedings if these plans are endorsed by your physician.

Your dietician will work with you regarding choices of food consistent with dietary plans arranged by your physician. Without monopolizing his or her time, try to develop a strategy that will maximize your caloric intake.

Special items such as elemental diets frequently do not arrive on the floor until ten o'clock in the morning. By working with the dietician, you should be able to arrange to have special foods of this type brought to the floor either earlier that day or possibly even the previous afternoon, so that you can begin your intake of calories early in the morning.

PHYSICIANS

If your hospital does not have a house staff (physicians in training, employed by the hospital), all your interactions will probably be with your personal physicians and the nursing staff. In hospitals with active teaching programs, there will be a group of house physicians and medical students participating actively in your care. A potential disadvantage is that multiple examinations may possibly tire you out, especially on the first day, when everyone will seem to be asking you the same questions over and over. Under these circumstances, it is perfectly acceptable to suggest to this group of physicians that some of the evaluations might be deferred until the next day. As part of an initial physical examination, a rectal examination is usually indicated. If you have severe perianal disease, and especially if your own physician has done a rectal examination, you should request that this part of the examination be omitted. A reasonable compromise is that only one rectal examination be done on the day of admission.

There are, of course, many advantages to having house staff and medical students participate in your care. One is that there are physicians available to you twenty-four hours a day who know your case in detail. The medical student in particular can be of great help to you, since he or she generally has more time to help explain things.

It is important that you communicate openly with your personal physician about your feelings and concerns. It is reasonable for you to know what routine is planned for you each day. Sometimes, in the crunch of a hectic work schedule, your physician might have overlooked some aspect of care that is important to you. Do not be afraid to point out these gaps, but at the same time be reasonable in your level of expectation.

TRAVELING WITHIN THE HOSPITAL

Traveling for diagnostic studies can be time consuming and frustrating. It is not unusual for patients to be kept waiting before, during, and after such tests, sometimes only for the next available transportation back to the room. This can sometimes take up the greater part of a day. If your strength does not permit you to sit up for long periods of time, insist on a stretcher rather than a wheelchair. Make sure that you bring extra socks and slippers, a bathrobe, and an extra blanket if needed. The ward clerk and nurse can help you with these details. You should understand, however, that at times waiting cannot be avoided if there are emergencies which take precedence. Always have a book, magazine, needlecraft, or some other form of entertainment with you!

If you find that you are really too weak to wait any longer, do not hesitate to alert either the ward clerk or a nurse in the area and ask that you be returned immediately to the floor. Be polite, but be firm.

YOUR MEDICATIONS AND TREATMENT

Learn something about intravenous therapy. For example,

keep an eye on the bottle itself. As the fluid level nears the bottom of the bottle, ring for the nurse to change bottles before it runs out. There is no danger to you at all if the intravenous fluid does run dry, or if a small amount of blood backs up into the tubing, but this may cause the intravenous needle to become clogged and the IV may have to be restarted in another place. This is sometimes painful and should be avoided if at all possible. If an IVAC pump is being utilized to provide intravenous fluids at a fixed rate, learn something about the use of this equipment at the bedside.

If your stomach must be kept deflated with a nasogastric tube that aspirates fluid and air into a suction bottle, learn something about this process. For example, prior to insertion of the nasogastric tube, make sure to specify which nostril is more open so that the tube will be less likely to irritate you as it is being inserted. You should also know that you may have a gagging sensation as the tube is being inserted. This can be overcome partially by sniffing air in through your nostrils. This has a tendency to counteract coughing and spasm in the back of your throat. Once the tube is inserted properly make sure that it is taped firmly in place with adhesive tape from the tube itself onto the bridge of your nose. If the tube is not secured firmly in place, it may become dislodged as you move in your sleep, and may even come out altogether. Make sure that the suction machine is plugged into the wall, that a light is flashing periodically indicating that the machine is on, and also note whether small amounts of fluid and air are actually being aspirated through the nasogastric tube into the transparent tubing that connects the tube to the receptacle. One good way to determine whether suction is satisfactory is to disconnect the nasogastric tube periodically from the plastic tube. When this takes place, there should be an audible hiss indicating that the suction is working properly.

Keep track of your input and output of fluids. It is important for your doctor to know how much urine you pass each day, and the volume of fluids you receive. You can keep track of this easily with a paper and pencil and do these measurements yourself.

One of the most important ways in which you can help your doctor is by keeping an accurate stool chart describing your bowel movements and the time they occur. This provides your doctor with an objective picture of your progress during the many hours he or she cannot be in the hospital. It will help in noting your response or lack of response to treatments.

LEAVING THE HOSPITAL

When the time comes for you to leave the hospital, your doctor may have detailed instructions he or she would like you to follow. If it is easier for you, you may request that these instructions be written down so that you will not forget them. Be sure to check with your doctor whether there are any limitations in diet or physical activity, especially if you have had surgery. Your doctor will probably schedule a follow-up visit in the office shortly after your discharge.

15

OBTAINING LIFE INSURANCE AND MEDICAL INSURANCE

For the individual with IBD or *any* chronic disease, obtaining insurance has always presented a maze of conflicting information and seemingly insurmountable obstacles. This need not be the case with life insurance, however, which is now available more readily than at any time in the past. Competition within the insurance industry, significant increases in employee benefits offered by employers, and the decreased stigmatization in our society toward individuals suffering from certain chronic medical conditions may each have contributed in some measure to the greater availability of life insurance coverage. The question now to consider is how to get the best possible coverage at the lowest possible rate.

LIFE INSURANCE COVERAGE

A recent survey of members of the Greater Boston Chapter

of the National Foundation for Ileitis & Colitis showed dramatically the variability which may exist in the life insurance coverage of IBD patients. Eighty percent of the respondents who reported owning life insurance were between 20 and 50 years old. The amount of insurance owned appears to be related to age, sex, and whether it is an individual or group policy. Other factors that may be involved in determining the amount of insurance available and the premiums paid are the length, severity, and type of IBD, and whether your agent has the ability to place coverage with a number of different carriers.

Forty percent of those answering the survey reported that they had trouble obtaining or keeping their insurance. The difficulties they encountered included the following:

- the imposition of ratings and surcharges resulting in higher initial and continuing premiums
- prolonged search for a company that would issue an acceptable policy
- the requirement of an extra medical exam
- the imposition of a waiting period
- the refusal of insurance when the disease is active or undiagnosed

GETTING AROUND THE OBSTACLES

IBD patients who responded to this survey represent a wide range of experiences from the very positive to the very negative. Since the insurance business is large, diverse, competitive, and based on complex principles, we sought advice from a number of insurance professionals on the question of how to minimize the difficulties met in obtaining insurance, and how to get the most comprehensive coverage for the insurance dollar. The following sections will outline the suggestions made by these representatives of the insurance industry. The discussion is general because the amount of insurance needed, the ability to pay, and the degree of risk presented to the insurance carrier will vary from individual to individual.

Group Life Insurance

This type of insurance is available in the fringe benefit programs offered by most corporations and institutions. The rates are determined by the actuarial evaluation of the group covered. The cost (if any) to the employee is quite low at the outset in comparison with most individual policies, although it may increase over time. The benefit is equal to, or a multiple of, your base salary. When the employee terminates employment with that group, he or she may usually convert the group coverage to individual coverage at his or her then attained age—which may involve a fairly high cost. Consequently, reliance solely on a group life insurance policy of this type is not recommended by our consultant.

In some situations, a type of quasi-group arrangement may provide an IBD patient with permanent life insurance at standard rates. An example of this arrangement is a pension or profit-sharing plan, in which a group of individuals, such as partners in a business or professional corporation, applies for insurance together as a unit. The carrier will agree to issue at standard rates an amount of insurance based on the number of lives, and will take the extra risk of including someone who would ordinarily be surcharged rather than losing the entire group.

Individual Life Insurance

Attempting to purchase individual life insurance shortly after the onset of IBD or during a flare-up usually results in a declination or heavy rating. Conversely, insurance purchased

147

before onset of illness (especially if the policy carries an option to purchase more coverage at the same or similarly favorable rates, i.e., a so-called guaranteed purchase option) is unaffected. Since IBD may involve more than one family member, these options may be particularly attractive to young people whose families have a history of IBD. When the IBD patient is symptom-free or the disease is under control for years, insurance can often be purchased at near standard rates, or a higher-rated policy may be re-evaluated and the premium reduced. Once a premium has been reduced, it cannot be raised again. This type of review should be conducted periodically to determine whether a person rated because of disease continues to be at impaired risk. Patients who are in remission should remember to request a re-evaluation of their rating every one to two years. If your disease is active, do not request review.

The Role of the Insurance Agent in Obtaining Life Insurance

"Don't shop around for an agent, make an agent shop around for you." This advice from the president of an employee benefits firm suggests that you should choose an agent on the basis of his or her knowledge of the insurance market rather than trying to poll a number of agents for the least expensive policy they can sell you at the time. The best agent will know which companies may be more aggressive in underwriting and more willing to take risks in a given economic climate, and will then be able to obtain the most favorable policy for you. The agent's knowledge or influence with a particular carrier can expedite a better deal for you.

In addition to the prospective agent's knowledge of the insurance industry in general, you should inquire what this includes regarding IBD. Many agents are not familiar with the disease, nor with the need for obtaining as much information about a client's medical condition as possible. Because a company cannot raise an initial premium once it is contracted, it will attempt to rate a client "for the long haul," according to a medical officer of one prominent life insurance company. The actual price of the insurance depends primarily on the age of the client and what the actuarial tables show about the life expectancy of people with IBD. Nonetheless, because of the competitive nature of the industry, companies are constantly studying the results of their own actuarial experiences, and individual companies may handle a given disease differently. Almost all carriers purchase reinsurance to reduce their losses from the insurance they sell to high-risk clients.

In purchasing life insurance, then, it is important to tell your doctor that there will be an insurance inquiry. Your physician's medical report will be the single most important piece of underwriting information to the insurance company. Because of issues of privacy, lack of understanding of the importance of their input, and inadequate reimbursement for the time taken to complete a difficult insurance query, many physicians may not provide enough relevant information for the agent to negotiate the best policy for you. Explaining this to the physician may help him or her write a report that is more favorable to you. Companies differ in the way an unusual report is viewed, and the more complete the record is, the more attention it will get from a senior officer with the ability to make nonroutine decisions on offering coverage.

MEDICAL INSURANCE COVERAGE

Most people in the United States obtain group medical insurance through their place of employment. This means that individuals with Crohn's disease or ulcerative colitis must be healthy enough to work, or must be covered as dependents under the health insurance policy of a family member. Several nonworking women with IBD in the Boston survey noted that they feared they would have trouble obtaining insurance on their own if they were not married. Even those who are working may find that the policy offered by their employer will not cover "pre-existing conditions" until after a full year of employment, or will cover them only after a fixed period of time during which they are "symptom-free" or "treatment-free."

It is also generally true that the larger the company or institution you work for, the more generous the medical coverage is likely to be, and, in most cases, the fewer the restrictions in covering persons with a chronic condition like IBD. This is because the liability of carrying a "high-risk" individual is spread over a large pool of employees. Conversely, a smaller company may offer a less comprehensive (and less expensive) medical insurance policy with more restrictions. If it is at all possible to choose, the individual with IBD who needs good medical coverage would do far better working with a large employer.

If no group plan is available to you at work, or if you are unemployed or unable to work, you will have a very difficult time obtaining medical coverage. While individual life insurance can usually be obtained at some cost, one insurance representative offered the option that IBD patients are "wasting their time" trying to get individual health insurance from a commercial carrier. If you find yourself in this situation, there are two other options you might explore. In some states, Blue Cross/Blue Shield offers an "open enrollment period" for a few weeks every year. During this time, they will accept applications for individual coverage from people desiring medical insurance. If this option is available in your state, you should take advantage of it even though the premium will be relatively high. It will be your only available medical coverage and it is always possible to convert to group coverage should you begin working again.

A second option you should explore is the group medical coverage frequently offered by fraternal organizations, clubs, national associations, etc. Because of their large membership, these organizations can sometimes offer low-cost group medical insurance to paid-up members. If you belong to such an organization, you may be able to obtain some medical coverage in this way.

Conversion to Individual Medical Coverage

If you are leaving employment and have not yet found your next job, find out if you can convert your group medical coverage to an individual plan for which you pay the premiums. If you can arrange for this type of conversion, pay your premiums promptly and regularly! If you allow your individual insurance to lapse, you may not be able to obtain coverage again unless you begin working again. In many instances, Blue Cross plans will not enforce restrictive "pre-existing conditions" clauses if your coverage with them has been continuous.

Coverage for minors under most Blue Cross plans expires when the child is 19. In some cases, the upper age limit is 23. At least a full year before the age limit is reached, parents of a child with IBD should begin inquiring about an individual policy in their son or daughter's name. This is especially important because IBD in young people is frequently more severe and disabling than in adults and many are unable to work and therefore to obtain medical benefits on their own. If the young IBD patient is a student in college, it may be several more years before he or she is ready for employment, and most student health plans do not have the breadth of coverage necessary for inflammatory bowel disease.

16

WHAT TO DO
IF YOU BECOME
DISABLED

SOCIAL SECURITY DISABILITY?

The Social Security Act, passed in 1935, originally paid retirement benefits only at age 62 or 65. The Social Security Administration later realized that workers disabled by illness before age 65 should be entitled to some compensation. Monthly disability benefits are tax-free, and are meant to replace a part of a family's lost earnings for as long as the worker's condition prevents *substantial gainful activity*.

No one is automatically entitled to these benefits. You must first apply. There are two basic questions to ask yourself before you apply for disability benefits:

1. *Are you insured?* Social Security Disability works like any other insurance plan. You must pay something into the system (Social Security taxes) to get something out. Under Social Security law, insured status means that you have worked at least twenty quarters out of the past forty (five

years out of the past ten years) prior to being disabled. These work periods need not be continuous.

In addition, you must not now be working. If you are, then, by definition, you are not eligible, even if you are seriously ill. You must generally be out of work for twelve months or more before applying, or there must be a likelihood that you will be out of work for at least twelve months. Even if you wait the full year, the benefits you receive if you are eligible will be retroactive.

2. *Are you suffering from a determinable condition?* You must have a *diagnosis* (e.g., Crohn's disease or ulcerative colitis) that is severe enough to limit significantly your ability to do work, and which is now preventing you from doing your former work.

The Social Security Administration has published a *Handbook for Physicians* that contains a "Listing of Impairments" (see below) to help physicians in making a disability evaluation. If it is determined, through detailed reports filled out by your doctor, that because of the severity of your disease you "meet the listing," then you are automatically entitled to receive benefits. (The listings below do not reflect the current use of the term *Crohn's disease* to include both granulomatous colitis and regional enteritis.)

5.06 CHRONIC ULCERATIVE OR GRANULOMATOUS COLITIS (demonstrated by endoscopy, barium enema, biopsy, or operative findings). With: A. Recurrent bloody stools documented on repeated examinations and anemia manifested by hematocrit (the ratio of red blood cells to whole blood) of 30 percent or less on repeated examinations; OR B. Persistent or recurrent systemic manifestations, such as arthritis, iritis, fever, or liver dysfunction, not attributable to other causes; OR C. Intermittent obstruction due to intractable abscess, fistula formation, or stenosis (stricture); OR D. Recurrences of findings of A, B, or C above after total colectomy; OR E. Weight loss as described under 5.08.

5.07 REGIONAL ENTERITIS (demonstrated by operative findings, barium studies, biopsy, or endoscopy). With: A. Persistent or recurrent intestinal obstruction evidenced by abdominal pain, distention, nausea, and vomiting and accompanied by stenotic areas of small bowel with proximal intestinal dilation; OR B. Persistent or recurrent systemic manifestations such as arthritis, iritis, fever, or liver dysfunction, not attributable to other causes; OR C. Intermittent obstruction due to intractable abscess or fistula formation; OR D. Weight loss as described under 5.08.

Even if you do not qualify automatically under the listing of impairments, you may still receive benefits. The question then becomes: What is the nature of the impairment, and how has it affected your residual functional capacity. Simply stated, this means determining whether, with the impairments you have, you can still do any productive work on a sustained daily basis. This is the area where most of the Social Security disability "battles" are fought, and where the services of a lawyer are usually needed.

You may apply for Social Security Disability in writing at any local Social Security office. This can often be a time-consuming and frustrating experience. It's a good thing to keep in mind that while the interviewer is taking information from you, he or she is also quietly evaluating your ability to sit or stand for long periods, the number of times you had to use the bathroom during the long interview, and the amount of pain (or lack of it) that you are experiencing. On the basis of this "silent" evaluation, this worker may write the words "no apparent impairment" on your application.

Next, your application reaches the Bureau of Disability

Determination in your state. There an initial determination is made, based on information supplied by you, and sent by your doctor or hospital. (In many instances, Social Security will hire a local doctor to examine you to verify the medical report.) This initial determination is made by a medical doctor and a lay disability analyst after your file is complete.

If your claim is denied, you must ask for reconsideration within sixty days. At this time you should submit further evidence to strengthen your claim. Experience has shown that without fresh evidence, your claim will be denied.

If this happens, you must request a hearing by an independent administrative law judge. This will generally occur seven to twelve months after you first filed your application. To this hearing you should bring any further evidence, oral or written, medical or vocational, to support your claim. It is at this point that you should have the services of a lawyer.

If you lose the hearing, you have the right to ask the Appeals Council to review the record of the hearing. You do not testify before the council. The Appeals Council does not generally reverse the ruling of the administrative law judge unless it is legally wrong or factually incorrect; in fact, their reversal rate is quite low.

Failing this, you may press for a court hearing in your state. The court has three options. It can either affirm the administrative law judge's decision, reverse that decision and grant benefits, or ask for a rehearing.

Your lawyer is in a position to help you with your disability claim if he or she knows:

- *all* your symptoms, complications and impairments
- *all* medications you are taking, including their side effects. (You must show reasonable compliance with medical regimens. You have a right to refuse controversial or high-risk treatments.)
- the effects of the disease on your emotional state

Your lawyer will want to know whether he or she can get a detailed medical report from your doctor (including lab reports, endoscopy, and X-ray reports, and detailed clinical information). *A flat statement by the doctor that you are disabled is absolutely inadequate.* The medical report must contain:

- the date you were first seen by your doctor
- the course of illness
- the frequency of visits
- your symptoms and complications
- whether you "meet the listing" and why

You and your lawyer should see that your doctor has a copy of the Listing of Impairments. If your doctor feels you cannot meet the listing, have him or her quantify what work you can and cannot perform. This report must be in language a judge can understand and should contain information such as:

- whether you are able to take public transportation to and from work
- whether you need to lie down for periods of time during the day
- whether you are prevented from doing any pulling, pushing, or lifting on the job
- how many times a day you must use the bathroom

Remember it is your burden (and your lawyer's) to prove your claim. You both must be able to enlist your doctor's help to do this. Experience has shown that the younger and more skilled you are, the harder you will have to fight to get Social Security disability benefits.

Certain other types of evidence can be submitted to the administrative law judge. When pain is a factor in disability (as it often is in Crohn's disease and ulcerative colitis), some lawyers have sent their clients for special thermography tests. These tests help to quantify pain and make it less subjective. Your lawyer might also advise you to have a vocational work-up and/or a psychological evaluation. Both of these tests can be used as quantifiable evidence of your inability to work.

Most lawyers handling Social Security Disability cases charge a modest retainer of $250, which is not refunded. If you lose your claim, all you have lost is the retainer. If you win, a process that may take eight to twelve months, your lawyer is entitled to the retainer plus no more than 25 percent of the past due benefits. This is subject to the approval of the Social Security Administration. Under the law, your lawyer may not take more than this amount.

What should you do if you have been receiving Social Security Disability benefits and are cut off? As of January 1982, disability benefits *must* be reviewed at least every three years, unless you are permanently disabled. During that three-year period, you must report:

- any changes in your condition (improvements)
- if you have returned to work. A nine-month trial work period is permitted as an incentive to return to work

If your benefits are cut off, you will be given an opportunity to appeal. Don't be discouraged. Twenty percent of people whose disability benefits are terminated never seek reinstatement of benefits. More than half of those who do can expect to win them back.

Dos and Don'ts about Applying for
Social Security Disability Benefits

Do keep records of your symptoms, medications, etc. to help your doctor write a detailed medical report for you.
Do have someone accompany you to the Social Security examining doctor to make notes and time the visit.
Don't be a martyr. If you are too sick to work, apply for

benefits.

Don't suggest to the Social Security office that no one would hire you, or that you can't get a job that pays enough. The test is not whether you can get a job but whether you can keep the job you have.

To contact an attorney in your area who can assist you in presenting your Social Security Disability claim, write or call:

National Association of Social Security Claimants'
    Representatives
P.O. Box 794
19 East Central Avenue
Pearl River, NY 10965
(914) 735-8812

Appendix

NFIC CHAPTERS

Chapters of the National Foundation for Ileitis & Colitis have been formed in many states. Each chapter is composed of a lay board and a medical advisory committee. Together, medical and lay leaders plan education seminars and fund raising activities for members and for the public at large. These activities increase awareness of inflammatory bowel disease and provide the funds urgently needed for research in IBD.

Chapters currently exist in the following states:

Arizona	Louisiana
California	Maryland
Connecticut	Massachusetts
District of Columbia	Michigan
Florida	Minnesota
Illinois	Missouri
Kansas	Nevada

New Jersey
New York
North Carolina
Ohio
Oklahoma
Pennsylvania

Rhode Island
Tennessee
Texas
Virginia
Washington

NFIC Offices: NFIC National Headquarters
295 Madison Avenue - Suite 519
New York, New York 10017
(212) 685-3440

NFIC Western Regional Office
12012 Wilshire Boulevard #201
Los Angeles, California 90025
(213) 826-8811

Greater New York Chapter
295 Madison Avenue - Suite 519
New York, New York 10017
(212) 679-1570

Ann Gorlitz South Florida Chapter
12550 Biscayne Boulevard
Suite 605
North Miami, Florida 33181
(305) 895-0617

Philadelphia Chapter
7718 Castor Avenue
Philadelphia, Pennsylvania 19152
(215) 742-1800

Greater Boston Chapter
1330 Beacon Street, Suite 320
Boston, Massachusetts 02146
(617) 734-3900

Houston Gulf Coast Chapter
2640 Fountainview
Suite 338
Houston, Texas 77057
(713) 783-0098

Michigan Chapter
17000 West Eight Mile Road
Suite LL 63A
Southfield, Michigan 48075
(313) 424-8656

Please call NFIC Headquarters for the address of the NFIC Chapter
nearest you.

Notes

CHAPTER 1

B. B. Crohn, L. Ginzburg, and G. D. Oppenheimer. "Regional Ileitis," *JAMA,*, 99(1932): 1323–9.

R. G. Farmer, and C. H. Brown. "Ulcerative Proctitis; Course and Prognosis," *Gastroenterology* 51(1966): 219.

J. H. Foley. "Ulcerative Proctitis," *New England Journal of Medicine,* 282(1970): 1362.

M. J. Goodman, and M. Sparberg. *Ulcerative Colitis* (New York: John Wiley & Sons, 1978).

H. Schachter, and J. B. Kirsner. *Crohn's Disease of the Gastrointestinal Tract* (New York: John Wiley & Sons, 1980).

CHAPTER 2

M. J. S. Langman. *The Epidemiology of Chronic Digestive Disease* (Chicago: Year Book, 1979), p. 139.
This short book has a 22-page chapter on "Chronic non-

specific inflammatory bowel disease" which is an excellent review of the world literature on the subject. There are 16 tables. Contained in only 3 paragraphs is a clear discussion of genetic factors in these diseases.

A. I. Mendeloff. "Epidemiology of Inflammatory Bowel Diseases," Chap. I in *Inflammatory Bowel Diseases*, J. B. Kirsner and R. A. Shorter, 2nd ed. (Philadelphia: Lea & Febiger, 1980).

This chapter of 20 pages describes the evolution of our understanding of IBD in epidemiological terms. It reviews what is known about ulcerative colitis and Crohn's disease as they affect different populations in different parts of the world. The author points out the pitfalls in carrying out epidemiological studies of these disorders, and the directions future studies should pursue.

A. I. Mendeloff, M. Monk, E. I. Siegel, and A. M. Lilienfeld. "Illness Experience and Life Stresses in Patients with Irritable Colon and with Ulcerative Colitis," *New England Journal of Medicine*, 282(1970): 14–17.

The psychological stresses and previous illnesses suffered by large numbers of persons with these two disorders are compared. The data show that persons suffering from the irritable colon seem more likely to show symptoms and to suffer from other diseases than do those with ulcerative colitis. The ulcerative colitis group in this study resembled the general population without ulcerative colitis, whereas the irritable colon group was definitely different. The possible problems in interpreting these data are extensively discussed.

CHAPTER 3

J. T. Sessions. "Inflammatory Bowel Disease," *Viewpoints of Digestive Diseases* 7(1973): 4.

W. R. Thayer. "Inflammatory Bowel Disease: Where are the frontiers?" *Medical Clinics of North America* 64(1980): 1221–31.

"Recent Approaches to Inflammatory Bowel Disease," *Practical Gastroenterology* 1(1977): 53–55.

CHAPTER 4

J. L. A. Roth. "Diagnosis and differential diagnosis of chronic ulcerative colitis and Crohn's disease," in *Inflammatory Bowel Disease,* ed. J. B. Kirsner and R. G. Shorter (Philadelphia: Lea & Febiger, 1980).

J. D. Waye. "Colitis, cancer and colonoscopy," *Medical Clinics of North America.* 62(1978): 211–24.

CHAPTER 5

A. J. Greenstein, H. D. Janowitz, and D. B. Sachar. "The extra-intestinal manifestations of Crohn's disease and ulcerative colitis," *Medicine,* 55(1976): 401–12.

F. Kern. "Extraintestinal complications," in *Inflammatory Bowel Disease,* ed. J. B. Kirsner and R. G. Shorter (Philadelphia: Lea & Febiger, 1980).

CHAPTER 6

L. J. Brandt, L. H. Bernstein, S. Boley, and M. S. Frank. "Metro-nidazole therapy for perianal Crohn's disease: A follow-up study," *Gastroenterology,* 83(1982): 383–7.

J. B. Kirsner, and M. J. Goodman. "The medical treatment of in-flammatory bowel disease," in *Inflammatory Bowel Disease,* ed. J. B. Kirsner and R. G. Shorter (Philadelphia: Lea & Febiger, 1980).

D. H. Present, B. I. Korelitz, N. Wisch, J. L. Glass, D. B. Sachar, and B. S. Pasternack. "Treatment of Crohn's disease with 6-mercaptopurine: A long-term, randomized, double-blind study," *New England Journal of Medicine,* 302(1980): 981–7.

R. W. Summers, D. M. Switz, J. T. Sessions, J. M. Becktel, W. R. Best, F. Kern, and J. W. Singleton. "National Cooperative Crohn's Disease Study: Results of drug treatment," *Gastroenterology,* 77(1979): 847–69.

CHAPTER 7

M. H. Floch. *Nutrition and Diet Therapy in Gastrointestinal Disease.* (New York: Plenum Medical Book Co., 1981).

R. J. Grand. "Malnutrition and inflammatory bowel disease," *The Advisory,* Greater Boston Chapter, National Foundation for Ileitis and Colitis (1979) vol. 1, no. 1.

D. H. Law. "Use of elemental diet and parenteral nutrition in patients with inflammatory bowel disease," in *Inflammatory Bowel Disease,* ed. J. F. Kirsner and R. G. Shorter (Philadelphia: Lea Febiger, 1980).

CHAPTER 8

D. J. Glotzer, and W. Silen. "The surgical approach to the treatment of chronic ulcerative colitis and Crohn's disease," in *Inflammatory Bowel Disease,* ed. J. B. Kirsner and R. G. Shorter, (Philadelphia: Lea & Febiger, 1980).

N. G. Kock, H. Myrvald, and L. O. Nilsson. "Progress report on the continent ileostomy," *World Journal of Surgery,* 4(1980): 143–8.

M.R. Lock, R. G. Farmer, V. W. Jagelman, I. C. Lavery, and F. L. Weakley. "Recurrence and reoperation for Crohn's disease: the rule of disease location in prognosis." *New England Journal of Medicine*, 304(1981): 1586–88.

A. G. Parks, and R. J. Nicholls. "Proctocolectomy without ileostomy for ulcerative colitis," *British Medical Journal,* 2(1978): 85–8.

A. G. Parks, R. J. Nicholls, and P. Belliveau. "Proctocolectomy with ileal reservoir and anal anastomosis," *British Journal of Surgery,* 67(1980): 533–8.

CHAPTER 9

A. J. Greenstein, D. B. Sachar, and A. Pucillo, et al. "Cancer in Crohn's disease after diversionary surgery," *American Journal of Surgery* 135(1978): 86–90.

D. B. Sachar, and A. J. Greenstein. "Cancer in ulcerative colitis: good news and bad news," *Annals of Internal Medicine* 95 (1981): 642–4.

W. R. Thayer. "Malignancy in inflammatory bowel disease," in *Inflammatory Bowel Disease,* ed. J. B. Kirsner and R. G. Shorter, (Philadelphia: Lea & Febiger, 1980).

CHAPTER 10

M. E. Ament. "Inflammatory disease of the colon: Ulcerative colitis and Crohn's colitis," *Pediatrics* 86(1975): 322–34.

E. J. Burbige, S. H. Huang, and T. M. Bayless. "Clinical manifestations of Crohn's disease in children and adolescents," *Pediatrics* 55(1975): 866–71.

R. J. Grand, and D. R. Homer. "Approaches of inflammatory bowel disease in childhood and adolescence," *Pediatric Clinic of North America* 22(1975): 835–50.

B. S. Kirschner, O. Voinchet, and I. H. Rosenberg. "Growth retardation in inflammatory bowel disease," *Gastroenterology* 75(1978): 504–11.

C. B. Lindsley, and J. G. Schaller. "Arthritis associated with inflammatory bowel disease in children," *Journal of Pediatrics* 84(1974): 16–20.

P. F. Whitington, H. V. Barnes, and T. M. Bayless. "Medical management of Crohn's disease in adolescence," *Gastroenterology* 72(1977): 1338–44.

CHAPTER 11

M. Mogadam, W. O. Dobbins, B. I. Korelitz, and S. W. Ahmed. "Pregnancy in inflammatory bowel disease: effect of sulfasalazine and corticosteroids on fetal outcome," *Gastroenterology* 80(1981): 72–6.

M. Mogadam, B. I. Korelitz, S. W. Ahmed, W. O. Dobbins III, and P. J. Baiocco. "The Course of Inflammatory Bowel Disease

During Pregnancy and Post Partum," *American Journal of Gastroenterology* 75(981): 265–9.

L. Zetzel. "Fertility, pregnancy, and idiopathic inflammatory bowel disease," in *Inflammatory Bowel Disease*, ed. J. B. Kirsner and R. G. Shorter (Philadelphia: Lea & Febiger, 1980).

CHAPTER 12

M. Mogadam, W. O. Dobbins, B. I. Korelitz, and S. W. Ahmed. "Pregnancy in inflammatory bowel disease: effect of sulfasalazine and corticosteroids on fetal outcome," *Gastroenterology* 80(1981): 72–6.

L. Zetzel. "Fertility, pregnancy, and idiopathic inflammatory bowel disease," in *Inflammatory Bowel Disease,* ed. J. B. Kirsner and R. G. Shorter (Philadelphia: Lea & Febiger, 1980).

CHAPTER 13

M. J. Goodman, and M. Sparberg. *Ulcerative Colitis* (New York: John Wiley & Sons, 1978).

J. E. Helzer, W. A. Stillings, S. Chammas, C. C. Norland, and D. H. Alpers. "A controlled study of the association between ulcerative colitis and psychiatric diagnoses," *Digestive Diseases and Sciences* 27(1982): 513–8.

P. R. Latimer. "Crohn's disease: a review of the psychological and social outcome," *Psychological Medicine* 8(1978): 649–56.

M. Monk, A. I. Mendeloff, C. I. Siegel, and A. Lilienfeld. "An epidemiological study of ulcerative colitis and regional enteritis in Baltimore, III: psychological and possible stress-precipitating factors," *Journal of Chronic Diseases* 22(1970): 565–788.

Glossary

abscess A localized collection of pus that may form in the abdominal cavity or in the rectal area in persons with Crohn's disease.

ACTH A hormone (adrenocorticotropic hormone) that can be given in injection form to stimulate the body's adrenal gland to release corticosteroids.

adenoma A tumor that arises from glands in the epithelial tissue (lining) of organs such as the colon.

adhesion The formation of fibrous bands or scars, usually following abdominal surgery, that may cause joining of exterior surfaces of the intestines. Adhesions themselves pose no danger and do not require surgical correction unless they cause an obstruction.

anastomosis The surgical creation of a passage between two organs. In IBD, for exam-

173

ple, after a segment of diseased bowel has been resected, an anastomosis is made joining the two ends of healthy bowel together. See also *resection*.

anemia   Lower-than-normal amounts of hemoglobin in the red cells of the blood.

ankylosing spondylitis   A chronic inflammatory disease of the spine and adjacent joints seen in some persons with Crohn's disease or ulcerative colitis. The disease overwhelmingly affects males, usually before age 30, and causes pain and stiffness in the joints of the spine, hips, neck, jaw, and rib cage. Occasionally, joints of the spine may become fused (ankylosis). Anti-inflammatory drugs, physical therapy, and occasionally surgery are used in treatment.

antibody   A protein substance produced by the body in response to the presence of some foreign protein or microorganism (antigen).

anticholinergic   A substance that temporarily blocks some of the nerves controlling intestinal contractions. Anticholinergics are used to control spasms of the bowel.

arthralgia   Pains in the joints, frequently experienced by persons with IBD.

arthritis   Inflammation of a joint, accompanied by pain, swelling, heat, or redness. In some cases there are structural changes.

azathioprine   An immunosuppressive drug sometimes used in the treatment of Crohn's disease that has not responded to other medications. This drug has been shown to be helpful in reducing or eliminating the dependence on corticosteroids in some patients. It is

174

	used occasionally in ulcerative colitis.
Azulfidine	See *sulfasalazine.*
barium enema	An X-ray examination of the colon and rectum after liquid barium has been infused through the rectum.
biopsy	A small piece of tissue taken from the body for examination under the microscope. A biopsy is taken by a special instrument attached to the endoscope during examination of the rectum, colon, stomach, etc. A biopsy is used to confirm the diagnosis of Crohn's disease or ulcerative colitis, or to check periodically for the possibility of cancer.
borborygmi	Characteristic rumbling sounds in the bowel caused by the passage of air through the intestine.
breath tests	Simple, painless tests which help detect lactose intolerance (absence of the enzyme needed to digest milk sugar) or bacterial overgrowth in the intestine.
bypass operation	A surgical rerouting of intestine so that intestinal contents bypass a diseased segment. Once the operation of choice in Crohn's disease, the bypass has been largely replaced by surgical resection of the diseased bowel. See also *resection.*
cecum	The first part of the large intestine which adjoins the last part of the small intestine (terminal ileum).
cholestyramine	A drug, taken by mouth, that helps to bind excessive amounts of bile acids in the intestine. These bile acids sometimes cause increased diarrhea in persons with Crohn's disease, especially after the removal of a portion of the terminal ileum.
clubbing	An abnormal shaping of the finger-

175

nails in some patients with Crohn's disease or ulcerative colitis.

colon The large intestine.

colectomy Surgical removal of the colon. See also *proctocolectomy.*

colonoscopy A test in which a flexible, lighted tube is inserted through the rectum to examine the colon. Biopsies may be taken as part of this test. Sedatives are usually given to make this procedure more tolerable.

continent ileostomy The surgical creation of an ileal pouch inside the lower abdomen to collect waste after colectomy for ulcerative colitis. No bag is required, and the pouch is emptied regularly with a small tube inserted through a nipple opening in the lower front part of the abdomen.

cortiscosteroids See *cortisone.*

cortisone An anti-inflammatory drug, part of a group of drugs known as glucocorticosteroids. Cortisone is used to reduce inflammation in Crohn's disease and ulcerative colitis, and may be taken by mouth in tablet form, intravenously, or through the rectum in enema, suppository, or foam preparations.

distal Farthest away from the trunk of the body. For example, the rectum is distal to the colon.

distention An uncomfortable swollen feeling in the abdomen often caused by excessive amounts of gas and fluid in the intestine. Distention may be a sign of intestinal obstruction.

duodenum The first third of small intestine through which food passes from the stomach.

dysplasia Alterations in the cells of the colon

176

seen under the microscope after biopsies have been performed. Severe dysplasia in IBD indicates that cancer cells may begin growing in the colon, and that surgery may be necessary.

edema Accumulation of excessive amounts of fluid in the tissues, resulting in swelling.

electrolyte A substance essential to body function that conducts an electric current when in solution. Sodium and potassium salts are examples of important electrolytes.

elemental diet A specially prepared liquid meal without residue containing all necessary nutrients. These preparations are used to help IBD patients gain weight and to rest the bowel.

endoscopy A general term for the examination through a lighted tube of any natural body opening. Types of endoscopy include gastroscopy, sigmoidoscopy, and colonoscopy.

erythema nodosum Red swellings occasionally seen on the lower legs during flare-ups of Crohn's disease and ulcerative colitis. These lesions are an indication that disease is active, and they usually subside without a trace when the disease is treated.

exacerbation An aggravation of symptoms or an increase in the activity of disease; a relapse.

febrile Running a fever. The presence of fever in a patient with IBD is an indication of increased disease activity.

fecal fat test A three-day measurement of the amount of fat in the stool (steatorrhea). Increased amounts of fat in the stool may indicate poor absorption in the small intestine.

fissure   A crack in the skin, usually in the area of the anus in Crohn's disease.

fistula   An abnormal channel occurring between two loops of intestine, or between the intestine and another structure such as the anus, bladder, vagina, or skin. Fistulas are more common in Crohn's disease than in ulcerative colitis.

Flagyl   See *metronidazole.*

flatulence   The passage of large amounts of gas through the rectum.

folic acid   One of the vitamins responsible for the maintenance of red blood cells. Folic acid deficiency may occur in IBD patients, especially in those taking sulfasalazine, and can be corrected by taking oral supplements of the vitamin.

gastroenterologist   A physician specially trained in the diagnosis and treatment of patients with gastrointestinal disease. Your local medical society can provide a list of gastroenterologists.

granulomas   Microscopic abnormalities characteristic of Crohn's disease.

granulomatous colitis   Another word for Crohn's disease of the colon or Crohn's colitis.

heartburn   A painful, burning sensation of the esophagus, usually felt in the chest.

hemorrhoids   Painful, dilated veins of the lower rectum and anus, seen as a complication in persons with IBD.

hyperalimentation   A means of supplying patients with additional nutritional support, either by nasogastric tube feedings or by peripheral intravenous infusion.

ileoanal anastomosis   A newer operation for ulcerative colitis in which the rectal tube is retained after colectomy. The innermost mucosal layer of the rectum is stripped off, and a pouch is made from ileum and attached directly above the anus. This preserves continence, and allows the patient to evacuate in the normal manner through the anus. This operation is also known as the "pull-through" or Parks operation.

ileocolitis Crohn's disease involving ileum and colon.

ileostomy The diversion of fecal waste through a surgically created opening of the ileum to the body wall. Waste collects in a bag attached to the skin by special adhesive.

ileum The lower third of small intestine which joins the large intestine (colon).

immunosuppressives Drugs which act to suppress the body's natural immune response to an antigen. In the treatment of inflammatory bowel disease, azathioprine and 6-mercaptopurine are examples of immunosuppressives.

Imuran See *azathioprine*.

incontinence In IBD, the inability to retain feces, usually because of rectal inflammation.

irritable bowel syndrome (IBS) Altered motility of the small and large intestine, causing diarrhea and abdominal discomfort. IBS is mistakenly called spastic colitis, though it does not cause inflammation of the colon and has no relationship to ulcerative colitis.

ischemia Lack of blood supply to an area of the body.

IVP Intravenous pyelogram, an X-ray examination of the kidneys, ureters, and bladder, obtained from intravenous injection of a dye.

jejunum The middle third of small intestine.

179

lactose intolerance	Decrease or absence of the enzyme *lactase,* which enables the small intestine to digest lactose (milk sugar). People with lactose intolerance experience diarrhea, abdominal discomfort, and gas after ingesting milk or milk products.
lactose tolerance test	A test involving the drinking of a liquid rich in milk sugar. Blood samples are then taken over a period of time to determine whether there is a deficiency in lactase.
leukocytosis	An increased number of white blood cells in circulation.
metronidazole	An antibiotic which may be helpful in treating fistulas in some patients with Crohn's disease.
mucosa	The inner lining of a body cavity, such as the lining of the colon.
mucus	A whitish substance produced by the intestine that may be found in the stool.
nasogastric (NG) tube	A thin, flexible tube passed through the nose or mouth into the stomach. The NG tube is necessary to aspirate fluids that collect in the stomach when the bowel is obstructed or after intestinal surgery.
obstruction	A blockage of the small or large intestine preventing the normal passage of intestinal contents. In Crohn's disease, obstruction may be caused by narrowing or spasm of the intestine. Signs of obstruction are vomiting, abdominal pain, and distention of the abdomen.
occult blood	Invisible blood in the stool, often an indication of disease activity. There are simple laboratory tests that can determine the presence of occult blood.
perforation	An abnormal opening in the bowel

180

wall that causes intestinal contents to enter the normally sterile abdominal cavity.

perianal Pertaining to the area around the anal opening that often becomes inflamed and irritated in persons with IBD.

peritonitis A complication of intestinal perforation that results in the inflammation of the abdominal cavity covering (peritoneum).

polyp A small growth protruding from the mucous membrane, for example, in the bowel. Polyps may be flat, raised, or attached by a stalk to the mucosal surface.

prednisone A form of cortisone given in tablet form to reduce the inflammation of Crohn's disease or ulcerative colitis.

proctitis Inflammation of the rectum.

proctosigmoiditis Inflammation of the rectum and the lower part of the colon (sigmoid).

proctocolectomy Surgical removal of the entire colon and rectum.

proximal Nearer to the trunk of the body. For example, the ileum is proximal to the colon.

Purinethol See *6-mercaptopurine.*

pyoderma gangrenosum A type of sore that sometimes occurs on the extremities of persons with ulcerative colitis or Crohn's disease.

regional enteritis Another name for Crohn's disease affecting the small intestine.

remission A lessening of symptoms and a return to good health.

resection Surgical removal of a diseased portion of intestine. Reattachment of the two ends of healthy bowel is called *anastomosis.*

sigmoid colon The S-shaped portion of the large intestine that is joined to the rectum.

sigmoidoscopy A test in which a lighted tube is passed through the rectum into the sigmoid

	colon. Biopsies may be taken through the sigmoidoscope. Sedation is not usually needed.
6-mercaptopurine (6-MP)	An immunosuppressive drug found to be useful in closing fistulas and in reducing or eliminating dependence on cortiscosteroids in some patients with Crohn's disease. It (6-MP) is also useful in some cases of ulcerative colitis.
SMA$_{12}$	A laboratory test that allows for the measurement of 12 blood chemistries from a single blood sample.
septic	Contaminated with microorganisms or their poisonous products (toxins).
small bowel	Small intestine.
steatorrhea	Abnormally large amounts of fat in the stool, usually the result of poor absorption in the small intestine in Crohn's disease.
stenosis	Narrowing or stricture of a cavity such as the intestine.
steroids	See *cortisone.*
stoma	Artificial opening on the exterior of the abdomen after ileostomy surgery. Feces empty into an appliance fitted over the stoma with special adhesive.
sulfasalazine	A medication combining a sulfa component with a drug in the aspirin family. Sulfasalazine is used in mild-to-moderate attacks of IBD and to maintain a remission. The drug is thought to be more effective when disease is in the colon rather than the ileum.
tenesmus	A persistent urge to empty the bowel, usually caused by inflammation of the rectum.
terminal ileum	The last part of small intestine which attaches directly to the cecum.

Glossary

total parenteral nutrition (TPN)   The intravenous infusion of all nutrients through a catheter placed in a large vein near the collar bone. TPN is used to insure adequate nutrition in severely ill or malnourished IBD patients, to rest the bowel, and to prepare poorly nourished patients for surgery.

toxic megacolon   Acute dilation of the colon in ulcerative colitis (or occasionally in Crohn's disease), which may lead to perforation.

universal ulcerative colitis   Ulcerative colitis involving the entire colon from cecum to rectum.

upper GI series   An X-ray examination of the esophagus, stomach, and duodenum performed in the fasting patient after the ingestion of liquid barium. The duration of the examination can be prolonged to allow for viewing of the entire small intestine, including the terminal ileum. the X-ray is then known as an upper GI series with small bowel follow-through.

Index

abdominal abcess, 90
abdominal pain, 29
adenomas, 42
amebiasis, 19
amebic dysentery of colon, 3
anaerobic bacteria, 22–23
anal fissure, 31, 91
anal skin tab, 30, 31
anastomosis
  ileonal, 94–96
  resection with, 85, 86 (fig.)
anemia, 129
ankylosing spondylitis, 48
antibiotics
  colitis related to, 4, 20, 33,
    127–28
  in inflammatory bowel dis-
    ease (IBD) therapy, 66–67
antibody, 20, 24
  anticolon, 25–26
  antigen complex, 26
anticholinergics, 68
antigen-antibody complex, 26

aphthous stomatitis, 49
apthous ulcers, 30
Aronson, M.D., 22
arthralgia, 47, 115–16
arthritis, as systemic complication, 46–48, 115–16
atropine, 68
azathioprine, 62–64, 122–23

bacteria
  in bowel disorders, 4, 19–20
    33
  inflammatory bowel dis-
    ease (IBD), 19–20, 22–23
  overgrowth of, 76, 78
barium enema X ray, 33–36
B-cell, 24
BCG vaccine, 70
Bean, R.H.D., 61
Bernstein, Leslie, 66
bile ducts, inflammation of, 50
bile salt, depletion of, 74–76,
  77–78

biopsy
    with colonoscopy, 38–39,
        104
    with sigmoidoscopy, 33, 104
blacks, risk factors among, 16
bowel cancer, 106
bowel disorders, 3–4, 19–20
    See also inflammatory bowel
        disease (IBD)
bowel resection, 85–87, 123–24
Broberger, O., 25
Brooke, Bryan, 62–63
bypass operation, 87, 88 (fig.)

campylobacter infection, 19,
    128
cancer
    bypass surgery and, 87
    and Crohn's disease, 10–11,
        105–6
    in older patient, 126
    and ulcerative colitis, 37, 98–
        99
        biological behavior in, 102
        incidence of, 99–101
        prognosis of, 104
        risk factors in, 101–103
        surveillance techniques for,
            42–43, 104–106
catheter, in parenteral feed-
    ings, 79
child patient
    caloric intake for, 114–15
    delayed maturation in, 115
    diagnostic tests for, 116–17
    growth retardation in, 30, 31,
        111–14
    nutrition and, 80, 114
    joint pains in, 115–16
    medical insurance for, 151

medications for, 117–18
    psychological support for,
        118, 119 (fig.)
    in school, 116
    surgery for, 118
    symptoms of, 109–11
cholangitis, 50
cholestyramine (Questran),
    68–69, 77, 78
clostridia, 4, 19–20, 32–33
codeine, 67, 68
coherin, 69
colitis
    antibiotic-related, 4, 20, 33,
        127–28
    ischemic, 127
    See also ulcerative colitis
colon
    cancer of, 37, 99–106
    colonoscopic examination
        of, 37–42
    Crohn's disease of, 9, 10, 83,
        86–87
    diverticular disease of, 128
    dysplasia in, 42–43
    inflammation of, 4
    X ray of, 33–37
colonoscopy
    biopsy with, 38–39, 104
    for cancer surveillance, 105
    preparation for, 40–41
    pros and cons of, 39–40
    visual capability of, 37–38,
        41–42
continent ileostomy, 92, 94
corticosteroids
    for child patient, 117–18
    commonly used, 59
    dose and duration of, 59–60
    efficacy of, 58–59

emotional impact of, 133
for older patient, 129
side effects of, 60–61
surgery and, 84
corticotropin (ACTH), 59
Crohn, Burrill B., 3, 8
Crohn's disease
of colon, 9, 83, 86–87
colorectal cancer and, 10–11,
105–6
definition of, 1, 3
diagnosis of, 9–10
family history of, 10, 17
fertility and, 120–21
first description of, 8–9
of ileum, 36, 50–51, 52, 74,
82–83, 86, 87
immunosuppressive therapy
for, 62–65
nutritional complications of,
74–77
treatment for, 77–81
onset of, 10
late, 129
surgery for, 82–91
symptoms of, 29, 30, 31
terminology of, 9
See also inflammatory bowel
disease (IBD)
cromolyn, 69–70
cytomegalic inclusion virus
(CMV), 20
cytotoxic cells, 24

depression, 133
diagnostic tests, 10
barium enema
X ray, 33–36
for child patient, 116–17
colonoscopy, 37–42

emotional impact of, 133
gastroscopy, 43
GI series, 36–37
hospitalization for, 142
in pregnancy, 123
preparation for, 140
sigmoidoscopy, 33
diarrhea
antibiotic-associated, 67
as diagnostic sign, 29
medications against, 67–69
diet
before colonoscopy, 40–41
elemental feedings in, 78
for fat reduction, 77, 80
for ileostomy patient, 80–81,
88
and inflammatory bowel disease (IBD) risk, 15
for lactase deficiency, 77, 80
with mild disease, 81
oxalate content and, 76
parenteral feedings in, 78–
80
in pregnancy, 124
before surgery, 84, 88
See also nutrients
dieticians, hospital, 140–41
diphenoxylate (Lomotil), 67, 68
disability benefits, 152–58
disease, retrospective study of,
12–13
diverticular disease, of colon,
128
dysplasia, 42–43, 104–6

E. histolytica, 3
elemental diet, 78, 84
enema
barium, 33–34, 35–36

tap water, 34–35, 40
environment, and inflammatory bowel disease (IBD) risk, 15–16
enzymes, 72
epidemiology, 12
erythema nodosum, 48
eye problems
reddening, 30
as systemic complication, 49

family
history, as risk factor, 10, 17–18
support function of, 134–35
fats, digestion of, 72
fertility, effects of Crohn's disease on, 120–21
fever, 29
fiberoptic colonoscope, 37–40
fingernails, clubbing of, 30
fistulas
defined, 8
as diagnostic sign, 9–10, 30, 31
diverticula and, 128
medication for, 66
surgical management of, 89–90, 91
5-aminosalicylic acid (5-ASA), 23, 56
folic acid deficiency, 32

gallstones, 50–51
Goodman, M.J., 133
gastrointestinal (GI) series, 36–37

gastroscopy, 43
Giardia lamblia, 3–4
giardiasis, 4
Ginzburg, Leon, 8
Gitnick, Gary, 22
granuloma, 9
granulomatous colitis. See Crohn's disease

health insurance, 149–51
hematocrit, 32
hemoglobin, 32
hemorrhoids, 31
home parenteral nutrition (HPN), 79
hospitalization
admission process in, 137–38
diagnostic tests during, 35, 140, 142
instructions on discharge from, 144
staff-patient relations during, 139–42
tips for comfort during, 139
treatment in, 142–44

IBD. See inflammatory bowel disease
ileitis. See Crohn's disease
ileoanal anastomosis, 94–95
ileocolostomy, with exclusion, 87, 88 (fig.)
ileostomy
continent, 92, 94
diet and, 80, 88
permanent, 87–88, 89 (fig.)
in pregnancy, 124
temporary, 88, 95

in total proctocolectomy, 91–92, 93 (fig.)
immune response
abnormal, 23–24, 25–27
lymphocytes and, 24–25
stimulation of, 70
immunosuppressive therapy
in Crohn's disease, 62–63
double blind study of, 63–64
precautions with, 64–65
in pregnancy, 122–23
in ulcerative colitis, 61–62, 65
inflammatory bowel disease (IBD)
causative agents in antibiotic use, 4, 20
bacteria, 19–20, 22–23
immune response, 23–24, 25–27
viruses, 20–22
in children. *See* child patient
definition of, 3
diagnosis of
diagnostic tests in, 33–42
laboratory tests in, 32
medical history in, 28
mimicking symptoms and, 3–5, 19, 32–33, 128
in older patients, 127–28
physical examination in, 31
warning signs and, 29–30
disability benefits and, 152–58

hospitalization for. *See* hospitalization
incidence of, 13–14
in later years, 125–26
life insurance coverage with, 145–49
medical coverage for, 149–51
nutrient malabsorption in, 72–76, 114
onset of, 16–17
late in life, 127–30
in pregnancy, 121
and pregnancy, 120–24
risk factors for, 13
diet, 15
environment, 15–16
family history, 10, 17–18
race, 16
stress and, 131–33
support systems in, 134–36
systemic complications of, 44–52
causes of, 45–46
incidence of, 45
See also specific disorder
treatment of, 55, 142–44
nutritional complications and, 76–77
See also medication; surgery
See also Crohn's disease; ulcerative colitis
intestinal cancer, Crohn's disease and, 106
intravenous pyelogram (IVP), 51
intravenous therapy, 142–43
iron deficiency, 32

irritable bowel syndrome (IBS),
1, 4–5, 131
ischemia, 127

jaundice, 50
Jews, risk factors among, 14
joint pain, 30, 46–47, 115–16

K-cell, 25, 26
kidney stones, 51, 76
Kock, Nils, 92
Korelitz, B.I., 64

laboratory tests, 32
lactase deficiency, 74, 77, 80
life insurance coverage
  agent role in, 148–49
  group, 147
  individual, 147–48
  obstacles to, 145–46
liver disease, as systemic complication, 49–51
liver function test, 32
loperamide (Imodium), 67, 68
lymphocytes
  in inflammatory bowel dis-
    ease (IBD), 25–26
  types of, 24–25

medical insurance, 149–51
medical students, role in hospital care, 141–42
medication, 22, 23
  administration of, 55–56
  antibiotics, 66–67
  anticholinergic, 68
  antidiarrheal, 67–68
  for child patient, 117–18
  cholestyramine, 68–69
  corticosteriods, 58–61

emotional impact of, 133
  during hospitalization, 138,
    140, 142–44
  immunosuppressives, 61–65
  metronidazole, 65–66
  during pregnancy, 121–23
  side effects of, 57–58, 60–61,
    64, 66, 68, 77
  sulfasalazine, 56–58
  unvalidated, 69–70
metronidazole (Flagyl), 22, 65–
  66, 91
Mitchell, D.N., 20, 22
mouth
  inflammation of, 49
  sores inside, 30
mucous colitis. See irritable
  bowel syndrome
Mutual Help groups, 135–36
mycobacteria, 23

nasogastric tube, 143
National Association of Social
  Security Claimants' Representatives, 158
National Cooperative Crohn's
  Disease Study (NCCDS), 63–
  64
National Foundation for Ileitis
  & Colitis (NFIC)
  chapters of, 161–62
  Mutual Help groups and,
    135–36
nausea, 29
nervous stomach. See irritable
  bowel syndrome
night sweats, 29
nursing staff, patient relations
  with, 139–40
nutrients

absorption process for, 72, 73 (fig.)
for child patient, 114–15
defined, 71
malabsorption of, 32, 51–52, 72–76, 114
See also diet

Oppenheimer, Gordon, D., 8
oxalate, excess, 76

pain, abdominal, 29
paraminosalicylic acid, 23
paregoric, 67
parenteral nutrition, 78–80, 84, 88
pediatric patient. *See* child patient
perianal region
symptoms in, 30, 31
treatment of, 91
peristalsis, 4
Perlmann, P., 25
photophobia, 49
physicians, patient relations with, 141–42
plasma cells, 24
plasmapheresis, 70
polyps, 41–42
prednisolone, 59
prednisone, 56, 77, 122
pregnant patient
course of disease in, 121
diagnostic tests for, 123
diet for, 124
with ileostomy, 124
medication for, 121–23
onset in, 121
stress on, 124
surgery for, 123–24

Present, D.H., 64
proctocolectomy, with ileostomy, 91–92, 93 (fig.)
propantheline, 68
pseudopolyp, 42
pyoderma, 48–49

race, as risk factor, 16
rectal cancer, 37
Crohn's disease and, 105–6
ulcerative colitis and, 98–105
rectal examination, 31
red bumps, 48
Rees, R.J., 20, 22
regional enteritis. *See* Crohn's disease
remission, in ulcerative colitis, 6–7
resection, 85–87, 123–24
retrospective study, for risk factors, 12–13

sacroileitis, 47–48
salmonella infection, 19
shigella, 4, 33
Shorter, Roy G., 25
sigmoidoscopy, 33, 34, 104
sinus tracts, 31
6-mercaptopurine (6-MP), 61, 64, 122–23
skin disorders, as systemic complication, 48–49
skin lesions, 30
Social Security Disability benefits, 152–58
Sparberg, M., 133
spastic colitis. *See* irritable bowel syndrome
steatorrhea, 74
steroids. *See* corticosteroids

stomatitis, 49
stool examination, 32, 33
stress
  on family, 134
  on patient, 132–33
    during pregnancy, 124
  in irritable bowel syndrome,
  5
sulfasalazine, 23, 56–58, 77,
  117, 122
surgery
  for abdominal abcess, 90
  bypass operations in, 87, 88
    (fig.)
  for child patient, 118
  complications after, 90–91
  for fistula management, 89–
    90, 91
  ileoanal anastomosis, 94–
    96
  ileostomy, 87–89
    continent, 92, 94
    in total proctocolectomy,
      91–92, 93 (fig.)
  in pregnancy, 123–24
  preparation for, 83–84
  reasons for, 82–83
  resection, 85–87

T-cells, 24
tenesmus, 5, 7
terminal ileitis. *See* Crohn's
  disease
total parenteral nutrition (TPN),
  78–80
tuberculosis, 19, 23

ulcerative colitis
  colorectal cancer and, 37,
    98–99
  biological behavior of,
    102–3
  incidence of, 98–100
  in older patients, 126
  prognosis of, 102
  risk factors for, 100–102
  surveillance for, 42–43,
    103–5
  course of, 6–7
  definition of, 1
  forms of, 5, 7–8
  immunosuppressive therapy
    for, 61–62, 65
  surgery for, 91–96
  symptoms of, 5–6, 29, 30, 31
  See also inflammatory bowel
    disease (IBD)
ulcerative proctitis, 1, 5, 7–8
ulcerative proctosigmoiditis, 5
ureter, blockage of, 51
Ursing, B.O., 66

vitamins
  absorption of, 72
  deficiency in, 32, 52, 74, 76,
    77
virus, as causative agent, 20–22
white cells, in immune response,
  24–25

X ray, with barium enema, 33–
  37